"Rachel Jones's book, birthed during the pandemic of the century, is filled with painful truths about the American healthcare system that sound the clarion call for change."

—JESSICA ZITTER, MD, author of *Extreme Measures*

"Urgent, powerful, healing. Nurses and doctors should read this book, but hospital administrators most of all. US healthcare has reached a crisis point where those who care for others need care themselves to recover from epidemic levels of burnout. *Grief on the Front Lines* shows how that caring work can and must be done."

—THERESA BROWN, PhD, RN, author of the
New York Times best seller *The Shift*

"*Grief on the Front Lines* is a clarion call for a more compassionate approach to medicine—not only for our patients, but for ourselves as medical professionals. Rachel Jones succeeds in her attempt to "fill the void" in challenging the medical establishment to acknowledge the grief we experience by routinely facing "the reality of death and dying" and to create a more humane working environment, strengthen necessary support systems, and remove barriers to mental health services. She explores innovative approaches to addressing the most common causes of grief and distress, while acknowledging the limits of self-care. *Grief on the Front Lines* inspires a vigorous response to the needs of an overextended and downtrodden healthcare workforce, particularly as we emerge from a devastating global pandemic."

—ANTHONY MAZZARELLI, MD, CEO of
Cooper University Health Care and co-author
of *Compassionomics*

"Honoring the experiences and attendant grief of healthcare workers, Rachel Jones provides well-sourced documentation of the events of the pandemic and provides a call to action to bring a more compassionate healthcare system into being."

—RANA AWDISH, MD, author of *In Shock*

"*Grief on the Front Lines* could be called *The Real Story Behind Healthcare.* Rachel Jones makes great effort to weave this story in which healthcare providers often become molded by the suffering they have been inspired to try to palliate or cure. She relies on research and personal narratives to place a human face on those called to serve others. This story is a call to action to ensure that we heal while healing others. May this book serve to inspire healing and reveal that we are never alone in the struggle. It's not only important to Pause at death, but also to Pause in the pursuit of healing and life."

—JONATHAN BARTELS, RN, innovator of the Medical Pause

"In *Grief on the Front Lines* Rachel Jones takes us into the lives of the remarkable men and women who stand with us at times of loss and death and brings their own pain to life. A harrowing and unforgettable book."

—MICHAEL SHAPIRO, professor of journalism, Columbia University

"Rachel Jones has made an invaluable contribution to the literature on trauma and loss. *Grief on the Front Lines* is a devastating account of the heavy emotional burden placed on healthcare workers and a powerful indictment of a system that fails to care for its own. Passionately researched and rendered with eloquence and humanity, Jones's book reminds us that healers also need to heal—in today's world more than ever—and that empathy and connectedness are the surest balms for a grieving heart."

—ALEX STONE, author of *Fooling Houdini*

"Frontline healthcare workers have always been expected to balance their personal lives with the emotional realities of comforting those facing life-threatening illness. Most providers in hospitals, from emergency rooms to intensive care units and nursing homes, face an onslaught of unrelenting suffering and death that today has become even more tragic in the presence of infectious disease. Very few can bear the massive burden of grief and trauma without life-changing consequences.

Grief on the Front Lines takes the reader through a sobering journey of the overwhelming conditions so many of these special people face dozens of times each day. For the rest of us, placing hearts of thanks on front lawns and banging pots and pans every night in praise of these tireless individuals is a powerful way to express our gratitude. Here is a superb overview of the state of palliative care that belongs on your 'must-read' list to really understand the experience of these heroes. It ultimately will support readers to become more empathic. The inescapable fact is that secondary trauma and crippling grief breaks hearts; with time and love as healers, tragedies can become fortunate blessings that open us to compassion and lovingkindness—the best antidote to the natural experience of loss."

—WILLIAM SPEAR, end-of-life educator, Fortunate Blessings Foundation, Second Response Initiative, and Care for the Caregiver Program

"Sobering, heartbreaking, and filled with hope, *Grief on the Front Lines* is a must-read not only for every doctor, administrator, and healthcare worker, but for everyone subject to illness and death. Pulling back the curtain on the avalanche of stress, violence, and grief in the field charged with our well-being, this book brings together revealing personal accounts, latest research, and culture-shifting resources available for those working in the healthcare system. It's a seed of a new paradigm we cannot afford to miss."

—VERA DE CHALAMBERT, MTS, religious scholar, writer, and spiritual storyteller

"Healthcare workers often carry deep emotional and spiritual wounds that are not visible and are sometimes left untended. *Grief on the Front Lines* provides a much-needed exploration of the effects of trauma and grief on the very people we rely on to help us heal. Rachel Jones gently explores these wounds and shares strategies that healthcare workers can employ to support their own healing and give them strength to continue their work. The book highlights a growing movement toward recognizing and addressing the human needs of healthcare workers and ensuring the well-being of these highly committed individuals. With stories from mental health professionals, trauma specialists, and hospice providers, these accounts of grief and healing offer hope for doctors and other healthcare workers who are struggling with the challenges of the profession."

—REV. DON CHATFIELD, PhD, Lead Pastor, All Souls Interfaith Gathering, Shelburne, Vermont

Grief

on the

Front Lines

RECKONING WITH TRAUMA, GRIEF, AND HUMANITY IN MODERN MEDICINE

RACHEL JONES

Foreword by
Danielle Ofri, MD, PhD

North Atlantic Books
Huichin, unceded Ohlone land
aka Berkeley, California

Published by
North Atlantic Books
Huichin, unceded Ohlone land
aka Berkeley, California

Cover art © gettyimages.com/Sandra M
Cover design by Jess Morphew
Book design by Happenstance Type-O-Rama

Printed in Canada

Grief on the Front Lines: Reckoning with Trauma, Grief, and Humanity in Modern Medicine is sponsored and published by North Atlantic Books, an educational nonprofit based in the unceded Ohlone land Huichin (aka Berkeley, CA), that collaborates with part-ners to develop cross-cultural perspectives, nurture holistic views of art, science, the humanities, and healing, and seed personal and global transformation by publishing work on the relationship of body, spirit, and nature.

North Atlantic Books' publications are distributed to the US trade and internationally by Penguin Random House Publishers Services. For further information, visit our website at www.northatlanticbooks.com.

Library of Congress Cataloging-in-Publication Data
Names: Jones, Rachel
Title: Grief on the front lines : reckoning with trauma, grief, and
    humanity in modern medicine / by Rachel Jones.
Description: Berkeley, California : North Atlantic Books, [2022] |
    "Perspectives from healthcare workers." | Includes bibliographical
    references and index.
Identifiers: LCCN 2021038721 (print) | LCCN 2021038722 (ebook) | ISBN
    9781623176402 (trade paperback) | ISBN 9781623176419 (ebook)
Subjects: LCSH: Psychic trauma. | Grief.
Classification: LCC RC480.5 .J662 2022 (print) | LCC RC480.5 (ebook) |
    DDC 616.85/21–dc23/eng/20211012
LC record available at https://lccn.loc.gov/2021038721
LC ebook record available at https://lccn.loc.gov/2021038722

1 2 3 4 5 6 7 8 9 MARQUIS 26 25 24 23 22

This book includes recycled material and material from well-managed forests. North Atlantic Books is committed to the protection of our environment. We print on recy-cled paper whenever possible and partner with printers who strive to use environmen-tally responsible practices.

With love for my parents,
who always encouraged my passion for reading
and desire to explore the world

And in deep gratitude to all those
whose lives and work
serve the health and well-being of others

Contents

Part I: Death and Trauma in Medicine

Part II: Rediscovering Medicine's Humanity

Part III: Changes in End-of-Life Care

Foreword

As a medical resident, I'd learned never to trust a quiet Sunday. The first code on the rehab floor fractured the peace. We raced as a threesome to the sixth floor, but as medical consult, I had to be in charge. Midway through that resuscitation, another code was called on the OB-GYN. I left my two colleagues and sprinted to the ninth floor. The frazzled OB-GYN resident described the situation to me. "The patient is thirty-two years old, healthy, thirty-six weeks pregnant. Came to our clinic three days ago with some nausea, a little vomiting, but she looked fine. Baby was fine too. We sent her home and she came back today with the same symptoms—a little nausea, not much else. But now we can't get a fetal heartbeat, and her blood pressure's dropping."

The patient was curled on her side, her pregnant belly ensconced between her elbows and her thighs. A thick black braid snaked down her back, tied with a slim blue ribbon. I curled my fingers around her wrist to feel her pulse; it was at least 120 beats per minute. Her pressure was 80/50.

"How are you feeling?" I asked the patient. She turned her head sluggishly away from me. The OB-GYN resident whispered to me, "We just told her about the baby a few minutes ago."

"Can I examine you," I asked, as gently as I could, "to make sure you are okay?"

"My body is fine," she whispered harshly. "It's my soul that is sick."

We whisked her upstairs to the medical ICU, treating her with aggressive fluids and antibiotics, but it was clear that we had to get that baby out, *stat.* The ICU bay became an impromptu Labor and Delivery suite, as we coaxed the patient through an excruciating—and excruciatingly somber—labor. It was sixty of the longest minutes I've ever lived through. After a final soul-sapping push, an oblong mass of baby emerged—ash gray. The body slipped into our gloved hands, landing with what felt like the heaviest thud. But it was only a whisper.

A silence layered over us, a sadness so pure and unadulterated that no one could move or breathe for the better part of a minute. We could only stare at this tiny gray ball in the middle of our little circle. It was as if this inanimate being managed to pull away the center pole of a tent, collapsing a canvas of sorrow upon everyone present.

But I still had to tend to our patient's urgent medical condition. I attempted to listen to her heart and lungs—what few sounds I could discern between her sobs. The nurse wept openly as she cleaned and wrapped the baby, tucking it into the arms of the mother, while I drew blood and made preparations for an emergent CT scan. The scan would ultimately reveal intestinal ischemia—dead gut—as the cause of her sepsis and hypotension, but we didn't know that at the time. I continued my medical evaluation of the mother, trying to figure out what was going on, but I couldn't bear to look into her face; the contortions of grief were so brutal and immediate.

I averted my eyes as we readied our patient to go to radiology. The nurse gently eased the blue bundle from her arms as her stretcher was wheeled out of the ICU to the CT suite. And then it was just me, the nurse, and the baby. The nurse sat down in the visitors' chair, holding the baby against her scrubs, and waited. Waited for someone to come take the baby. I didn't know who it was who came to take away dead babies, or what happens to the dead babies. And I didn't want to stay to find out.

❦

Healthcare workers experience trauma and grief at all levels of training, yet these experiences are often only tangentially examined. Even in terrifying and intense situations, we often—as I did—back out of the room rather than confront the pain. We hastily get on with our work, stuffing the difficult emotions into the pockets of our white coats.

The COVID-19 pandemic was a crash course in trauma. Every possible emotion was packed into a concentrated moment. There was more death than many practitioners had ever experienced. Playing out simultaneously on a global and on a local scale, the drumbeat of pain and suffering was relentless. There was no respite, even when you hung up your N95 for the day, as you had to watch your workday experiences play out on the nightly news. Even those observing from the sidelines were not immune.

Grief on the Front Lines could not be better timed. A generation of healthcare workers in training have had their professional identities forged in a crucible of grief. These emotions, though, are not limited to pandemics and other crises. They occur throughout the lives and careers of medical professionals, often with accumulated effect. Emotions untended and unchecked can lead to frustration, burnout, medical errors, and even post-traumatic stress disorder (PTSD).

Death and loss are woven into the fabric of our daily work; if we didn't want to face this, we would have chosen careers safely ensconced in offices and spreadsheets. But we've chosen work that brings us into some of the most intimate and vulnerable moments of peoples' lives. While there are definitely moments of joy, healthcare workers experience grief and loss to an exceptional degree. At our more composed moments, we recognize the honor and fulfillment of being able to be at our patients' sides during these difficult experiences. But in the quiet of our thoughts, we grapple with these painful moments, reliving and re-suffering.

Years later, I still think about that baby. When I experienced labor and delivery of my own, I thought about that mother, travailing through the same agony but greeted at the other end by such profound sadness. I never spoke to anyone about that night in the ICU—not to my team, not to my supervisors, not to my friends. I didn't even recognize it as a grief that was worthy of time and acknowledgment. I wish now that I'd stayed with the nurse and the baby. I wish we could have cried it out for however long it took. I wish I could have reconnected with the patient to see how she fared in the weeks and months that followed.

Instead, I backed out of the room.

Hopefully this book will allow you to stay in the room.

Danielle Ofri, MD, PhD
Bellevue Hospital
New York City

Introduction
Facing Our Mortality

For as long as I can remember, I've been interested in death and dying and in how we humans treat each other. I've long found death intriguing—after all, what is it?—while suffering affects me deeply. When I was growing up, my family didn't have a television, and I recoiled in horror when exposed to violent local news stories, images of Hiroshima after the bomb, or advertisements seeking to support starving children in far-flung countries. *How,* I would wonder, *did we get here?*

Later, in my undergraduate sociology studies, that question prompted my thesis—a comparative analysis of the genocides in Rwanda and in Bosnia. My research only left me with more questions, but I felt strongly that a lack of media attention had contributed and was determined to become a journalist. After obtaining an MS from Columbia University's Graduate School of Journalism, I made a beeline for Venezuela, where I spent more than four years as a reporter. It was a couple of years in before I began to question my impact. Was I really helping people to understand each other, to explore viewpoints other than their own? Or, by reporting on the most contentious aspects of both sides of the political spectrum, was I only contributing to conflict? Eventually, I stopped, and returned to the US, where I took a job at the Downtown Oakland YMCA—one I felt certain would benefit the well-being of those around me.

Toward the end of my time in Venezuela, I stumbled across a life-changing article written by journalist Kira Salak called "Places of Darkness: Africa's Mountain Gorillas and the War in Congo." Published in *National Geographic Adventure* in 2004, the story explored the complex, ongoing conflict in eastern Congo. My revelation came in the form of

Father Jo, a bespectacled Belgian priest who had managed to retain his humanity in the midst of the terror. He told her: "People here believe they will be killed, and so they do the same thing to others that they're afraid others will do to them." *That's it,* I thought. *That's how we get here—how we do these things to each other. We're scared of our own deaths.*

Psychiatrist Elisabeth Kübler-Ross, in her revolutionary 1969 book *On Death and Dying: What the Dying Have to Teach Doctors, Nurses, Clergy and Their Own Families,* reached a similar conclusion. "Groups of people," she wrote, "from street gangs to nations, may use their group identity to express their fear of being destroyed by attacking and destroying others. Is war perhaps nothing else but a need to face death, to conquer and master it, to come out of it alive—a peculiar form of denial of our own mortality?" Drawing on her famous, and controversial, seminars at the University of Chicago Medical School, Kübler-Ross emphasized the need for clinicians to face terminal illness and death in order to better serve their patients. At the time, it was common for physicians not to tell patients that they were terminally ill or dying, and both doctors and nurses responded with anger and defensiveness when Kübler-Ross broached the subject. "Doctors who need denial themselves will find it in their patients," she wrote. "Those who can talk about the terminal illness will find their patients better able to face and acknowledge it."

Kübler-Ross is widely credited with promoting the hospice movement and nurturing a growing understanding of what it means to die well. More recently, access to palliative care has grown exponentially across the US, though some states, populations, and rural areas remain underserved. While much attention has focused on how clinicians' acceptance of death improves patient care, there has been little recent discussion of the impact on doctors, nurses, EMTs, hospice workers, and other healthcare staff whose patients suffer from chronic and terminal illnesses or traumatic accidents. Without denial, what do they have? Do they experience grief when a patient they've connected with is diagnosed with a deadly disease? How do they feel when forced to perform CPR on a ninety-year-old woman with stage-four cancer who, if she survives, will only suffer more? What is it like to witness suffering and dying in hospice every day? When bombarded with the additional stressors of workplace violence, bullying, moral distress, and health disparities, how do people cope?

I was able to explore some of these questions when, as a staff writer for SevenPonds, a small but determined end-of-life website whose editors' strength of character and tenacity to serve I never cease to admire, I had the opportunity to interview healthcare workers for an article about the traumatic nature of code blues in hospitals. Several I spoke with expressed gratitude. One woman cried throughout the interview: "I'm an emotional person," she said without apology. It seemed that the more doctors, nurses, and others were able to acknowledge their grief and face the reality of death and dying, the more they were able to connect with their patients, the less stress they experienced, and the more resilience they exhibited. This despite challenging work environments, minimal resources to support them, and limited literature dealing with death and trauma in healthcare—and even less related to grief.

This book attempts to help fill that void, while bringing all of us to a deeper understanding of our shared humanity and mortality. Sigmund Freud believed that humans are unable to conceive of their own deaths; recent evidence supports that. In 2019, a small study by researchers at Bar-Ilan University in Israel found a "self-specific neurophysiological death-denial index" in our brains, which makes it easier for us to associate death with the faces of strangers than our own, suggesting that we may be hardwired to fear and deny the possibility of our own deaths. It's no wonder, then, that our demise may be hard for us to imagine. "Whenever we attempt to do so, we can perceive that we are in fact still present as spectators," Freud wrote.

That may be, but by acknowledging the grief and trauma experienced by healthcare workers, we can implement programs and develop systems to support them. By addressing the difficulties around death and dying as a larger community, we can, perhaps, move closer. After all, we're all in this together.

Part I

Death and Trauma in Medicine

1

Fall from Innocence

We rarely go gentle into that good night.

—SHERWIN NULAND

Every year, tens of thousands of aspiring doctors, nurses, and other healthcare professionals immerse themselves in US educational and training programs, eagerly preparing for their roles as healers. In Pennsylvania in the 1980s, Rosalind Kaplan was one of them. And, like many others, she was sometimes shocked by the emotional impact of the traumas she encountered—gunshot wounds, stabbings, failed resuscitations. She vividly recalls one night as a resident on the hematology/oncology service when an elderly, extremely weak patient receiving chemotherapy experienced a massive gastrointestinal bleed; she had to perform CPR on him as he was bleeding out in the radiology suite. "He died alone, on a cold metal table, and I started imagining what that would be like," she said. Kaplan showed up to morning rounds in blood- and stool-coated scrubs, and when she began telling the attending physician what had happened, she started to cry. Later, the attending called Kaplan into her office to discuss the fact that she was having trouble dealing with death—an accusation Kaplan found absurd. "If I hadn't been upset I would have thought that was a much bigger problem," she said.

For medical students and residents, traumatic patient encounters begin during long, grueling days of training: four years of medical school—traditionally including two years of clinical work—followed by three to seven years of residency. In addition to facing death and trauma, students often experience massive workloads, long clinical hours, high expectations, and toxic work environments—which can cause depression, anxiety, and other serious symptoms. Meanwhile, they have little opportunity to process traumatic outcomes, to engage in self-care—or sometimes, even to sleep. One commonly cited satirical novel about a medical residency program—*The House of God*, by Samuel Shem—provides a harrowing account of a cynical resident exhibiting burnout, disconnection, and a callous lack of humanity. Its narrator embraces a sexist and ageist gaze, referring to a female administrator as a "large-breasted adolescent" and to elderly patients as "gomers"—an acronym for "get out of my emergency room."

A nursing degree, which typically requires two to four years of study, brings its own unique challenges that can also have damaging repercussions. Nursing students have reported excessive workloads and informational overwhelm that result in serious emotional, physical, and behavioral symptoms ranging from nausea to depression (a 2018 analysis of twenty-seven cross-sectional studies found that roughly a third of nursing students experience depression worldwide). In the clinical setting, students commonly experience performance anxiety, as well as feelings of inadequacy and a lack of confidence in decision-making. Negative or unsupportive relationships with faculty has been identified as a major stressor—one with far-reaching impact, as caring faculty plays a significant role in students' intent to graduate.

While schedules may ease following training, healthcare workers' challenges are far from over. Forty-four percent of US physicians feel burned out even when there's not a pandemic, according to Medscape's National Physician Burnout, Depression & Suicide Report 2019. Nearly a quarter of

ICU nurses develop post-traumatic stress disorder (PTSD), while studies have shown that both nurses and emergency medical technicians have a significantly higher suicide rate than the rest of the population. An estimated three hundred to four hundred physicians in the US commit suicide every year—the highest rate of any profession, according to one analysis.

These statistics are sobering, and the reasons for them are varied and complex. Many factors, for example, contribute to physician burnout—including bureaucracy, long work hours, and a lack of respect from colleagues or staff. Although little research has been done on the impact of grief or trauma, a 2017 study containing a small group of Canadian oncologists found that they experienced difficulty with the deaths of their patients, particularly those they considered young, long-term, or unexpected. The bedrock for this study came from previous research, which found that oncologists demonstrated sadness, crying, and loss of sleep, along with feelings of powerlessness, self-doubt, guilt, and failure.

Leeat Granek, a critical health psychologist and associate professor at York University in Toronto who co-authored both of the studies, said she was inspired to initiate the research after her mother died of metastatic breast cancer. "I knew I was feeling something," said Granek, whose mother had received treatment from her healthcare team for nearly twenty years. "And I found myself wondering, what's going on for them?" Granek found that in addition to regular feelings of grief, oncologists reported that they often felt responsible. "There's kind of this intellectual understanding that yes, you did everything that you could," Granek said. "But emotionally the feeling is, I'm supposed to cure this patient and they died. And I feel like a terrible failure that they didn't make it."

Granek said it's essential for healthcare systems to begin normalizing and validating feelings of grief and loss among practitioners. As the US healthcare system has developed into an increasingly corporate, insurance-driven model, many clinicians report feeling disconnected from patients and colleagues, a lack of autonomy in decision-making, insufficient support when dealing with workplace violence or bullying and other major challenges. When combined with an inability to process grief and trauma, healthcare workers can become overwhelmed—causing them to resort to negative coping mechanisms, leave the profession, or even commit suicide. "Acknowledgment would remove the stigma from the individual person and recognize that it's part of the work that people do," Granek said of grief. "People still feel shamed by it—they feel that they're alone, they still feel like they're the only one. It's not part of the ongoing conversation or training that they're getting from an early stage. So recognizing it on a structural, institutional, educational level would take all of that [off the shoulders of] the individual and put it back into the work, into the whole structure."

Sherry Lynn Jones, a former paramedic and ER nurse with a PhD in education, came to a similar conclusion regarding trauma. Jones was inspired to become a first responder by the firefighter-paramedic duo on the NBC television show *Emergency!* "We have expectations as paramedics that we're going to go out there and be Roy and Johnny and make a difference," said Jones, who started at as an EMS volunteer in her small Michigan town in the late 1980s, serving community members she often knew personally. "We're not trained in how to handle it when things go wrong."

Jones, who has since authored a series of books titled *Confessions of a Trauma Junkie*, still remembers the calls that had the biggest impact on her. There was the father who died during her first full code as a medic. There was a little boy who "went to pieces" when a car hit him on the road. And the teen who'd drowned—Jones, unable to bear the sight of his vacant, fish-like eyes, had stared down at her tennis shoes as she held his cold leg, trying to will the life back into him. Then there was a young girl, a friend of her daughter's, who lived across the street and died in a house fire. The ten-year-old had gone to alert her grandmother, then hid in a closet; by the time Jones, who wasn't working but hurried over to help, saw her, the girl's tender giggle and sparkling eyes were gone, replaced by an empty, soot-stained corpse. "I can still feel them," she said. "I still smell the smoke."

Early on in her career, Jones began working with the International Critical Incident Stress Foundation, doing stress management interventions with people in emergency services. "Because we also gave them information about preparedness and education, they did not respond so badly after that," Jones said. "You can inform and educate, and people know that these things are going to happen, and it's not such a big surprise." Jones continued to pursue her interest in education as it related to nursing, completing a doctoral dissertation for Walden University in 2016 titled "Nurses' Occupational Trauma Exposure, Resilience, and Coping Education." Her research confirmed that there is still a significant lack of formal training related to grief, trauma, and *resilience*—which psychologists define as the ability to adapt when facing adversity, trauma, and other forms of stress. "Resilience is not inherent with everyone, but it can be taught and it can be enhanced," she said. "That's where education is key."

Kristen Bunge, an ER nurse, said that a class on death and grief at Samuel Merritt University in Oakland helped expose her to the concepts— particularly as her professor, who'd led the class for two decades, lost her husband during the first week of the course. "She would wear sunglasses because she would break down crying," Bunge said. "Seeing firsthand someone who was going through so much grief—and this is someone who had taught this class for so many years—it's easier said than done." After five years as an ER nurse at multiple Los Angeles hospitals, Bunge splits her time between two hospitals in Pasadena and Santa Clarita. "I still learn to this day" about handling grief, said Bunge, who takes comfort from Buddhist principles around death and dying. "Coming to grips with some of those bigger ideas made it easier in my job to understand that it's just a part of life." Still, it's not always easy. "It can be so hard watching families go through this," she said. "I've got families kind of bringing me into their inner circle—this very private inner circle that you become a part of. And unfortunately sometimes you hear through the chain: 'Oh that person from yesterday passed away,' or 'Oh, they extubated that one and they didn't make it.' So it is hard. You kind of have to build up a mental wall when it comes to loss and death and grief."

"A Surreal Experience"

For many physicians-in-training, their first encounter with death in a medical context comes when dissecting a cadaver in anatomy lab. Justin Key, who studied at Mount Sinai's Icahn School of Medicine in New York, said that his class spent a fair amount of time reflecting on what it meant to handle a human body. "The school had a memorial service, where some people sang songs, and I read a little piece that I wrote that talked about honoring the people that donated their bodies," Key said. Initially, the cadaver's hands and face were covered, and dissection began with the back and spinal cord before working around to the front. The face remained covered until the very end—when Key's group turned their body over, they discovered an elderly white man with a full face that had been smushed to one side, likely due to how he'd been stored. "We quietly exchanged sad looks," said Key, whose brown eyes usually reflect his genuine smile. "It felt more real in some way."

While Key found working on a human body to be a "surreal experience," he said that because they were doing so every day, the experience quickly became normalized. His first encounters with death in internal medicine were, however, much more shocking.

One case that greatly impacted him as an intern was that of a male patient of around fifty years with an inguinal hernia that had blocked his ureter, causing kidney failure. The patient had delayed seeking medical attention for several months and arrived at the hospital badly in need of dialysis. The next day, Key went downstairs to where the patient had been staying while waiting for a bed, with the senior resident on rounds. They spoke with the patient, who was receiving dialysis, and obtained his permission for a blood transfusion to offset his low hemoglobin before heading back up to the seventh floor. Shortly after they got there, the code pager went off. It was their patient.

Key and the resident rushed back down to find him at the center of a code blue—laid out, with his shirt open, and the staff performing chest compressions. As a first-year resident, Key was expected to perform CPR, which he found especially draining due to the short rotation. "I just remember handling this person that I had just spoken to, and the violence of pushing, doing chest compressions," Key said. "And when I wasn't giving chest compressions, just going over to the side and trying to wrap my head around what was going on from an emotional standpoint, from a physical standpoint." Key said that the team tried to keep the code going until the patient's family could arrive, but ended up calling the time of death at around fifty minutes. "After that I took a second off to myself," Key said, who watched the family—a wife or sister, and some teenaged children—crying and consoling each other in the hall after meeting with the attending. "It had that feeling of suddenness to it," he said.

Very little research has explored the impact of patient deaths on physicians. Between 2000 and 2001, a small study of third-year medical students in the US found that 57 percent rated the experience of a patient's death as highly emotionally powerful. Two years later, a separate study of physicians, residents, and interns from two US teaching hospitals found that a third of doctors echoed the same description, while 23 percent of their peers disagreed, labeling patient deaths as highly disturbing instead.

Key found talking with colleagues after such situations to be helpful when processing his emotions. Typically, a team will gather after a code blue to debrief—either immediately after the event, or later for a more formal discussion. "I had a really good [senior] resident in terms of decompressing and talking about it," Key said. "But the nature of the hospital is that you have to move on. Once you go into the next patient's room, they don't know any of that, and it's not right to burden them with any of that."

In addition to life-threatening emergencies, many doctors-in-training find the everyday challenges presented by patients with serious illness to be emotionally strenuous. Danielle Verghese, an internal medicine intern at Thomas Jefferson University Hospital in Philadelphia, said that she struggles to find outlets for emotions such as grief—particularly when she finds her professional life intersecting with her personal life. Having recently lost an uncle to head and neck cancer, Verghese found herself deeply affected by a patient in her oncology clinic suffering from the same disease. "I was struck by feelings of grief and taken back to that moment looking at my uncle as his face underwent all those changes from radiation and chemotherapy," she said. Treatment can turn a patient's skin pink, red, or very dark, or cause it to blister and peel. "But there's no form for me to really process that as I'm sitting with a patient who's going through their own personal tragedy," she said.

Verghese said she also grapples with other negative emotions, particularly frustration. And while her frustration is caused by multiple factors—such as being unable to help someone who is chronically ill, or facing aggression from a suffering patient, or being overworked—Verghese finds it difficult to locate an appropriate outlet. In the residents' lounge, Verghese said, people will often congregate to vent their irritation about patients, staff, or other issues. "In some ways it's good because you're at least getting it out—you're not bottling it up, you're not internalizing it," she said. "But on the other hand, it also has this almost additive effect, where you start propagating this downward spiral." Rather than indulging in the negativity, Verghese has found that turning to family members—particularly her sister and cousin, who are also in medicine—can give her the perspective she needs. "For people who are first generation physicians, people who are the only ones in their friend and family circles who are taking this on, I really wonder how they manage to make it through," Verghese said. "We don't have too many healthy ways of processing these emotions."

"Don't Let the Titanic Sink"

When it comes to medical training, death and grief are often just the tip of the iceberg. Medical schools and residency programs are notorious for their ability to overwork students, build stress, institutionalize mistreatment, and reduce personal lives to shambles. Students and residents are immersed in what's commonly known as the *hidden curriculum*, a term coined by education researcher Philip Jackson in 1968 to describe the observation that schools not only impart explicit skills and content but also implicit lessons about what kind of behavior is accepted and valued. In medical education, examples can include the concept that it's acceptable to berate nonphysician staff; that surgery is too difficult for women; that doctors don't need proper food and sleep, or to express their emotions; or that some specialties are better than others. Many students and residents are subjected to a form of teaching known as *pimping*—rapid-fire questioning, often in front of their peers (such as, "What role do prostaglandins play in homeostasis?" or "What are the three signs of Charcot's triad?"), that can leave them feeling battered and even cause them to be shunned if they perform poorly. According to the Association of American Medical Colleges (AAMC), 40 percent of medical students experience some form of mistreatment, such as public humiliation or being subjected to negative or offensive behavior. While about a quarter report such behavior, of those, less than 40 percent are satisfied or very satisfied with the outcome. Students who are yelled at, cursed at, or who suffer other demeaning behaviors often go on to become physicians who themselves repeat the cycle of abuse.

Marginalized groups are more likely to experience such mistreatment. A study of AAMC data on mistreatment of US medical students graduating in 2016 and 2017, published in *JAMA Internal Medicine* in 2020, found that 35.5 percent reported experiencing at least one type of mistreatment, the majority of these being female (40.9 percent vs. 25.2 percent male); an underrepresented minority, Asian, or biracial (more than 30 percent each vs. 24 percent white); and lesbian, gay, or bisexual (43.5 percent vs. 23.6 percent heterosexual). While women now graduate from medical school at a rate nearly equal to men, they still experience unwanted sexual advances, limited maternity leave, and gender-based discrimination—not so far as one might hope from the accounts detailed in Joan Cassell's 1998 classic, *The Woman in the Surgeon's Body*, in which a male surgeon screams of his incoming resident: "Anybody but the girl! Give me a trained monkey—I'd rather have anybody but the girl!"

Racial discrimination, meanwhile, can include being denied opportunities for training or rewards; being subjected to racially/ethnically offensive remarks or names; and receiving lower grades or evaluations for race-based reasons. Those who endure such treatment have little recourse. Despite the fact that Abraar Karan was president of his class during medical school, he still felt unable to challenge multiple racist comments from his superiors, such as one professor who told him: "Abraar, Ahmed . . . it's all the same." As he wrote in a 2020 article for Boston's WBUR public radio: "He would be writing my evaluation, and I could choose to either brush it off, or risk hurting my career."

The effects of such a culture are devastating. Studies have shown that medical students and residents experience greater depression, emotional exhaustion, depersonalization, fatigue, and burnout when compared to US college graduates from other disciplines. The American Medical Student Association (AMSA) has reported that medical students are three times more likely to commit suicide than their peers in other academic commitments, while an analysis of medical residency deaths conducted between 2000 and 2014 (published in *Academic Medicine*) supported this when discovering suicide as the top cause of death for male residents, and second-highest for female residents.

Alison Cesarz was in her fourth year at Rush Medical College in Chicago when the long hours, pressure of making major life decisions, and loneliness of being separated from her friends on clinical rotation began to take its toll. Usually an active person who valued community, Cesarz's blonde locks and sensitive eyes took on a dull hue as she began to lose interest in eating, socializing, her long-term boyfriend, and even running—one of her favorite hobbies. She broke up with her partner. She was losing weight, fantasizing about jumping off her building's third-floor balcony, and binge drinking "as a way to kind of avoid the pain." Still, Cesarz wasn't compelled to take action until she was matched with her dream program—a psychiatry residency at the University of California San Diego (UCSD).

"I realized that, 'I want to do a good job, and right now I don't feel able,'" Cesarz said. "And also, 'I'm going to move away from all my support.' Those thoughts were really scary to me, and that's when I think I told my mom and my roommate." Cesarz's family and friends were supportive, and once she began taking an antidepressant and receiving therapy, her outlook improved dramatically. "When you talk about it, you actually experience relief," said Cesarz, who set up therapy through her residency program prior to moving to California. "And that it doesn't necessarily define you." Cesarz said that UCSD provides resources such as the Healer Education Assessment and Referral (HEAR) program, which makes two therapists available via instant message through a confidential computer system and accommodates her therapy hours. She also attends weekly ninety-minute process groups with her class, during which residents' clinical hours are covered and an outside therapist facilitates the discussion to ensure confidentiality. It's something Cesarz would like to see made available "to all specialties, and medical students as well"—as she would have benefited from the services during her schooling, and many other programs fail to provide similar options.

More than a quarter of physicians-in-training experience depression or depressive symptoms, according to studies published in the *Journal of the American Medical Association (JAMA)*. Srijan Sen, the Frances and Kenneth Eisenberg Professor of Depression and Neurosciences at the University of Michigan's Depression Center, has found that roughly half of first-year residents, or interns, are depressed—up from nearly 42 percent in 2007–2009. "It's been a problem for a long time," said Sen, who nods his smooth-shaven head to emphasize his point. Sen was depressed during his training, watched his colleagues struggle, and had close friends who committed suicide. "It's difficult to discuss mental health issues and struggles, and so, oftentimes, the people who are struggling don't reveal it to anyone else, and everything seems to be okay until the tragedy happens," he said. Even those who successfully complete their programs can bear scars: many absorb the driven, self-harming work ethic exemplified in medical training, while others adopt callous, maladaptive behaviors modeled by superiors.

Sen, who's been analyzing first-year residents for more than a decade through his Intern Health Study, has found that they are more likely to experience depression in programs containing poor faculty feedback and inpatient learning opportunities, long work hours, and superior institutional research rankings. In addition, women are more likely to suffer depression than men, partly because they tend to feel more torn over family obligations. "Making sure the workload is manageable is important," said Sen, who considers fifty to fifty-five hours a week a reasonable range and suggests that institutions reduce the burden on residents by hiring staff to input data, answer phones, transport patients, or complete other nonmedical tasks. "People working eighty hours a week are much, much more depressed than the people working seventy hours a week, while those working one hundred hours a week are almost all depressed." Sen added that there are ways to structure shifts that can promote better sleep. "People who are sleeping less are definitely more depressed and also more likely to make medical errors, so getting adequate sleep is critical both for the physicians and the patients that they treat," he said.

Since 2003, the Accreditation Council for Graduate Medical Education (ACGME) has limited work hours for all residents to no more than eighty per week. This policy also restricted consecutive work hours to twenty-four, with the caveat of extending four additional hours for necessary transition purposes. Still, those who work overtime often under-report to keep their programs running smoothly. During her intern year in family medicine at the University of Pittsburgh Medical Center, Frances Southwick, now an osteopathic family medicine doctor practicing in California, regularly failed to report hours above the weekly maximum. "I felt behind, and I wanted to prove that I cared, and it was still never enough, no matter how many hours I stayed up," said Southwick, who authored a book about her experience called *Prognosis: Poor: One Doctor's Personal Account of the Beauty and the Perils of Modern Medical Training*. Southwick was used to being a high performer and struggled with not having grades—a tangible marker of how she was doing—or significant feedback from superiors. She budgeted her time, scheduling just ten to twenty minutes a day to spend with her wife, Jude, and over-thought small decisions such as what to eat, avoiding salad because it took too much energy to chew. On her surgical rotations, she battled with how to respond to questions like "Are you married?" which, if she revealed her sexual orientation, could either result in a relatively positive reaction, or in being ignored for the rest of the week. Her pixie-like frame suffered from the lack of sleep—perhaps more than most, as she was later diagnosed with narcolepsy—and she found herself dozing off during menial tasks, or even experiencing visual, and sometimes auditory, hallucinations. She had started taking an antidepressant, but it had limited effect, and she didn't know what else to do. The breaking point came after Southwick overheard her supervisor complaining about her performance. The next morning, Southwick wrote a suicide note and drove herself to the 40th Street bridge, where—if her supervisor hadn't called—she very well could have jumped. "I just couldn't see a way forward," she said.

Since making it through and authoring her book, Southwick has become an advocate for reshaping the system. She's formed an interdisciplinary committee of therapists, physicians, social workers, pre-med students, medical students, and residents from institutions around the country to draft a set of recommendations. These include mandatory monthly meetings with a confidential therapist, or time spent in alternative self-care such as yoga, tai chi, or qi gong; one weekday per month for residents to handle personal healthcare, car repair, and other basic needs; and six weeks of paid time off a year. "The training process has to change," said Southwick, adding that while many programs are now bringing in consultants to teach self-care, the current structure doesn't really support that. "To me, that's like watching people flounder after the *Titanic*, and saying, 'Just give them a back rub while they're drowning, wouldn't that be nice?' And it's like, no—give them a life raft. Don't let the *Titanic* sink."

Sneaking the Peanut M&M

The concept of self-care has been taking hold in medicine. In 2016, the World Medical Association (WMA) created an international workgroup consisting of members from different cultural, religious, and racial backgrounds to analyze the Declaration of Geneva. The document—a modern-day version of the 2,500-year-old Hippocratic Oath, to which most physicians pledge their allegiance upon completion of medical school— was adopted in 1948 and hadn't been revised in a decade. Drawing on nearly two years of surveys and other feedback from national medical associations, external experts, and public consultations, the committee decided to incorporate a new clause on physician well-being. The revised declaration, adopted by the WMA General Assembly on October 14, 2017, includes the statement: "I will attend to my own health, well-being and abilities in order to provide care of the highest standard."

Granek said this change represents an important cultural shift in the mindset of the healthcare profession. "In there, there's a kind of acknowledgment that you must take care of yourself, and that there are these really challenging aspects of practicing medicine that require support," she said. Still, acknowledging the need for self-care and creating the space and opportunities to benefit from it are two different things. Many doctors-in-training report that despite the availability of some services, such as group meetings, to deal with the more difficult aspects of their jobs, they find themselves unable or unwilling to participate. And finding time for personal self-care practices—or even to maintain a healthy lifestyle—can be nearly impossible for students and residents who are adhering to strict rotation schedules, putting in long hours of study, and spending nights on call, as well as for medical professionals with more challenging schedules.

Key, in his third year of residency for psychiatry at the Semel Institute for Neuroscience at the University of California, Los Angeles, said that due to the program's mental health focus, there's a strong emphasis on mental health for practitioners. Residents are encouraged to receive personal therapy, and after Key lost a patient who was in her thirties to a pulmonary embolism, the school expedited services for him. "That was really hard—she was kind of young, and I was thinking about whether there was anything I could have done better or faster," Key said. Meanwhile, he struggles with the knowledge that some of his outpatient clients could choose to commit suicide. He sees the therapist every Monday "to decompress a lot of the things that happen." In addition to therapy, Key draws on his spirituality in difficult situations such as resuscitations. "I pray, or try to be mindful, or think about God's presence there," he said. "Just think about the things that are out of my control, so I can better [perform my] role."

Verghese said that while she appreciates the cultural change in language, she simply doesn't have the time to incorporate self-care into her own routine. "People are happy to talk about wellness, they're happy to talk about resources and getting connected to resources," she said. "I think the next phase is to actually manifest these resources." In Verghese's residency program, there isn't a therapist who specifically addresses the needs of medical students and residents—unlike the program in which a friend of hers is enrolled. "They mandatorily speak to a psychiatrist at least once in the year," Verghese said. "And that's a nice way of taking away the stigma of mental healthcare and kind of normalizing the process of going to see a therapist, going to see a psychiatrist, and managing your own mental health in a preventative and not just a reactionary way."

Verghese added that her residency program incorporates a wellness week that includes lectures on exercise, nutrition, and art therapy—"all of which are well-intentioned efforts, but they didn't really acknowledge the constraints that we work in." One of the therapist's suggestions was to take a day off. "There's no way I can take a day off from work," Verghese said. "They were telling us about all these things that we should be doing—you know, eat these foods. Sleep like this. Work out like that. All things that I already know that I should be doing, and it just kind of compounds and highlights the fact that I can't do that right now." Instead, Verghese said she would appreciate "more candid conversations about what we're going through"—including how to deal with death, or how to prioritize self-care, such as advice on carving out a short time for exercise, or packing one healthier meal. "Those, I think, would be really helpful because they acknowledge the difficulty while providing a positive take on it," she said.

For many healthcare workers, such as bedside nurses, long hours and rare breaks are a challenge that extends throughout their careers. Jones, who spent eleven years as an ER nurse at a Michigan hospital as well as two in Nevada, said that her patient load was often overwhelming. "I've had seventeen patients in a day," said Jones, who didn't take breaks and could rarely find time to go to the bathroom or sneak a peanut M&M from the "clean" pocket of her scrub jacket. "I've had horrors that I had to just walk away from and go on to the next person who's crying because they didn't get a warm blanket and ice water when you were doing CPR three beds away." After a particularly challenging day, Jones said she'd make popcorn, eat a peanut butter-and-jelly sandwich, and watch mindless television. "You're too tired to make a healthy meal, which is what would be best," Jones said. "Sometimes you're so exhausted that you can't even get to sleep, much less maintain sleep. And then you go back and you do it again the next day."

Still, Jones found the work strangely satisfying. Once, the family of the man who had been her first code when she was working as a medic ended up in her ER, and Jones overheard his wife pointing her out to her daughter as "the nice paramedic who tried to help your daddy." Jones was incredibly touched. "It still gives me goose bumps to this day," she said. "At the end of many days, you come out and say, this wasn't possible but I did it. And you remember and count the blessings of the people in whose lives you made a difference." Jones added that making use of "gallows humor," as well as focusing on positive outcomes with colleagues or through journaling, helped her to get through the more stressful times.

Even nurses working in less trying circumstances grapple with challenging supervisors, difficult emotions around death and dying, and maintaining a positive work-life balance. Chris Poole, who after ten years as an acute care nurse maintains an aura of unflappable calm, works on the medical-surgical floor at the University of California, San Francisco (UCSF), assisting patients undergoing surgery for mostly gastrointestinal issues. Poole considers himself highly fortunate to work at a California hospital, where state law not only limits nurse-patient ratios, but also mandates a break nurse, so that staff can actually take time to sit down. Still, early on Poole had worked with a particularly abrasive nurse practitioner who sometimes put him down and made him question himself. "When you're getting bullied or you're feeling disrespected or not valued, it's super distressing—it gets at the core of who you are," Poole said. "So I would have sleepless nights." He also experiences difficult emotions around some patients, such as the fifty-year-old woman with inoperable, metastasized cancer with her children in tow. "It can bring tears to your eyes, and these patients can stay with you," said Poole, who often connects with people over the course of his twelve-hour shift. "It's probably not the healthiest thing, but there's a lot [of emotion] there under the surface."

Like many healthcare workers, Poole relies mostly on personal outlets to process such challenges, such as biking and swimming. He said that exercise has helped him to maintain a positive mental state, as well as to prepare for the physical demands of his job. He finds spending time with his family therapeutic, while domestic duties help him establish a routine. Poole will sometimes discuss particularly difficult cases with his mother, who was also a nurse, but acknowledges that other means of processing would be helpful. "It would probably be good for me to do journaling or talk about it in a group, and I don't do any of that," Poole said. While there are some support groups available to nurses at UCSF, Poole said that because he lives about forty minutes away in Berkeley, he wouldn't attend on his days off. "I'm sure it would be good to get together with other nurses and talk, because we all experience this," he said. "But most of us never talk about it."

In her research, Granek found that this was common. "Everybody's feeling the same way, and saying the same things, but they're not talking to each other," Granek said. A 2017 study of oncologists in both Israel and Canada revealed that the top desire for these specialty physicians coping with terminal patient illnesses was simply the validation of their grief and other related emotions. Such acknowledgment would easily and drastically prevent burnout. In addition, they also expressed interest in lectures, seminars, trainings, group debriefings, and most importantly, the opportunity to take time off. "There's a huge variation in terms of what people found helpful in coping with these emotions," Granek said, who advises that institutions provide a range of interventions and make these offerings opt-out rather than opt-in to normalize their necessity.

Sen has also found that doctors—both in training and beyond—typically feel that they're alone in struggling and suggests that team leaders address this by revealing their own challenges. "One thing that seems to be really effective is when senior leadership and physicians talk about their own problems," Sen said. "So if the residency program director, or department chair, or head of the hospital is willing to say that I got depressed during my training, or I struggle with depression, or I oftentimes have anxiety about whether I did the right thing with this patient, and are able to talk about it openly, that normalizes it for everyone else."

In more than five years, Kristen Bunge, the ER nurse in California, said she's rarely found herself discussing the emotional aspect of her work with anyone besides her parents or boyfriend. Doing so, she said, would probably help prevent her from becoming callous to patient deaths, which she often witnesses intimately at the bedside. "There are times when somebody comes in and passes away, and there are no family members there, and it's kind of like working on a machine," Bunge said. "You kind of have to pull back to that emotional aspect of: this is a human being." Bunge has developed her own practices to remain connected and will typically sit with a patient who doesn't have anyone else present when they die. "Whether they're cognizant of it or not," Bunge said. "Just kind of hold their hand as the heart monitor goes down. Let [the patient] know they're not alone."

Bunge said she'd find therapy helpful, but although her hospitals make it available, the hours are limited and "nobody ever uses it because nobody really knows how to access it." The one time she really felt a real outpouring of support—not only from the hospital, but also from the larger community—was when a student at nearby Saugus High School pulled a gun and opened fire on others in the courtyard. Four of them, including the shooter, ended up at her hospital, where three later died. "When it comes to kids it's a whole other story," Bunge said. "That hits you real hard." Afterward, the hospital bought the nursing staff lunch, and students wrote thank you cards voicing their support. The nurses were given time to sit down and eat together, and they opened up about their feelings during their morning huddle. "It was kind of nice to talk about it, to heal," said Bunge, who'd like to see easier access to therapy and more regular debriefings. "Because I think people carry more than they know."

Training programs for doctors, nurses, and other healthcare workers provide minimal education on dealing with such tragedies, while immersing students in demanding environments that stretch their mental and physical capacities to the limit. Doctors-in-training are often hazed and mistreated, are socialized into a callous culture, and experience high rates of depression. Some students are faulted for showing emotion; others hide their anxiety and depression; almost all struggle to eat and sleep well; and many develop maladaptive thought and behavioral patterns. While some programs—particularly those in psychiatry—provide better access to mental health services, and many are embracing a growing acknowledgment of the need for self-care and emotional processing, students remain constrained by long hours and heavy workloads—challenges that, for many, extend throughout their careers. Freshly minted doctors and nurses may emerge from training with the appropriate medical knowledge, but they are also often drained and beaten down. And many feel ill-equipped for the emotional challenges of the work—including tough conversations with patients and families, and traumatic patient losses.

2

The Nature of Grief

Every surgeon carries about him a little cemetery, in which from
time to time he goes to pray.

—RENÉ LERICHE

Patricia Numann, the first female surgeon to join SUNY Upstate Medical
University's faculty in 1970, had long been familiar with death. As a young
child, she visited family members' graves and gathered wildflowers for a
neighbor's post-mortem viewing; in high school, she lost three friends and
neighbors to a tragic car accident; and in medical school, she took time
off to care for her mother who was dying of pancreatic cancer. She studied people with terminal diagnoses and sat on the committee that formed
hospice in Syracuse. Even so, there were several patient deaths in her more
than thirty-five-year career that were harder than others to take.

"There were a couple that will stand out until I die," Numann said, recalling a forty-two-year-old man with a rare blood clotting disorder who'd died
on the operating table, and whose son sought her out years later for advice
on the same condition. It was rare for a death to occur in the operating

room, and when it did, it affected Numann deeply—particularly if the patient was young. "I had two children in a row die in the operating room after trauma, and that was very, very challenging," she said. One boy had been in a car accident and hadn't been wearing his seatbelt; the second had been hit by a car while riding his bicycle. Numann, who was in residency at the time, called in her co-resident to take over. "He came in and covered for me, and I went home for a while," she said. "Because I knew if it happened a third time I was done. I didn't know that I could go back."

Grief can be defined as the neuropsychobiological response to significant loss, often involving distress, separation anxiety, confusion, regret, and other strong emotions. Everybody experiences grief differently, and its length and quality vary depending on the individuals and circumstances involved. Doctors, nurses, paramedics, and others who work closely with illness and death have to find their own ways to navigate and process occupational grief while remaining as available as possible to the needs of their patients. And depending on their individual makeup, their work and home environments, their support systems and other factors, this exposure can, over time, profoundly affect their mental and emotional well-being.

Often, grief is not a short-term experience: Years later, medical professionals retain vivid memories of the deaths that touched them most. For some, it's changed the way they practice. For others, it's caused them to reflect on their own lives, or to develop more efficient ways of coping. Some practitioners have refined their communication skills with acutely, chronically, or terminally ill patients, while medical training and other programs have developed ways to assist them in sharing bad news more effectively. Meanwhile, healthcare workers in underserved communities who witness the impact of social determinants of health and racial discrimination on their patients have been motivated to advocate on their behalf, grieving their patients' circumstances while pushing for better living conditions; improved access to early-stage medical care; curricula that educates clinicians on relevant social issues; and more racial diversity in the workforce.

For healthcare workers in any role, the commonality is this: grief is a burden they must bear.

Patients Who Get into Your Heart

Most medical professionals have experienced patient deaths that are, for whatever reason, exceptionally heart-wrenching. Sometimes it's because the patient was young; sometimes because the death was unexpected; sometimes because the patient reminded them of someone they love. These situations can profoundly impact healthcare workers, forcing them to develop more effective coping strategies, affecting their relationships, and bleeding into other aspects of their personal lives. For both patients and providers, finding closure often helps to mitigate the stress, and diverse approaches can include attending funerals; avoiding funerals; saying goodbye; journaling; sharing case notes; and helping patients and their families make hard decisions.

For Don Dizon, the director of women's cancers at Lifespan Cancer Institute and director of medical oncology at Rhode Island Hospital, the deaths that most affect him are "the ones that should never have happened"—such as the 16-year-old with ovarian cancer who only lived to see her eighteenth birthday, or the mother diagnosed with ovarian cancer three months after she gave birth. "They absolutely change you," Dizon said. "Each time someone gets into your heart you find out: How can I construct a better wall so that I'm still standing five years from now?" Oncologists build relationships with patients—and often, their extended families—over time, making a balance between healthy empathy and clinical distance especially challenging. "You get invited to special moments in their lives that have nothing to do with their cancer," said Dizon, who has watched patients outlive their children, suffer through divorces, attend children's weddings, or witness the birth of their grandchildren. "It's such a profound thing when you hope for the best and it doesn't happen."

While Dizon attended the funerals of both the previously mentioned women, the new mother's stayed with him for months, and he determined shortly after the eighteen-year-old's that he wouldn't participate in any more patient memorials. "It's something I've discovered that I need to do to persevere and to sort of go beyond the grief so I can see the next person," he said. Instead, Dizon now brings his stylish, soft-spoken presence to the bedside as he bids farewell to those who are moving into home hospice or approaching death in the hospital. "I'll let them know that it was a tremendous honor to be in their lives and to get to know them and their family," he said. Clinicians typically take comfort from having some form of farewell: some may do so by attending patient funerals; others, like Dizon, prefer to find closure at the bedside.

Janine Overcash, a geriatric nurse practitioner and professor of clinical nursing at The Ohio State University who's spent most of her career in oncology, said that she finds herself considering the welfare of patients she sees every couple of weeks for treatment long after their visits. "I often think, 'I wonder if they got home okay, I know they were really tired,'" she said. "You know when their daughters are visiting and you wonder how things went." Overcash takes comfort in minor improvements, such as when changing medications means someone's not nauseous anymore and they're able to achieve a small goal such as visiting someone. Despite forming attachments, Overcash, who has also worked as a nurse in ICUs, in a burn unit, in trauma, and in hospice, typically finds long-anticipated deaths easier to process than those that come suddenly—including young people with "terrible brain cancers" or who've suffered traumatic accidents. "It changed the way I parented," said Overcash, who had two sons of her own and raised a third. She strongly discouraged all three from going on motorcycles, riding horseback, or sitting in the backs of moving pickups. "You look at risks as very real," she said.

The fact that patient deaths affect clinicians differently depending on things such as age and parental status is something that Alexandra Jabr, a paramedic educator in the Los Angeles area of California with a master's in mental health specializing in grief and bereavement, has often witnessed in the field. Jabr spent about fifteen years as an active paramedic and now teaches aspiring paramedics in community colleges and counsels fire departments on occupational resilience, behavioral health, and death communication. "The way I respond to a child dying is different from the way a parent is going to respond," Jabr said. Instead,

Jabr found herself reacting strongly to a young couple who'd suffered a car accident in which the husband died and his wife waited for hours on the side of the road. "It was heartbreaking because we were the same age," Jabr said. "It was just the association that changed for me, and I never quite forgot that."

Sometimes, medical staff find themselves engaged in difficult clinical work while mourning personal losses, a situation that can prove exceptionally demanding. Once, Numann was performing an operation when she was informed that her sister had died. Fortunately, her partner had happened to scrub in with her, and was able to take over while she stepped outside. "I walked out and cried," Numann said. "And I told the patient afterwards what had happened."

For Jennifer Caputo-Seidler, an internal medicine physician and assistant professor at the University of South Florida's College of Medicine, her worst day as a doctor occurred on the anniversary of her father's death, when she was a senior resident in the ICU. "I was already in an emotional headspace, but as trainees there's no backup," Caputo-Seidler said. At 6 a.m. she showed up in her usual scrubs to be confronted with a patient who'd had an elective procedure the previous day, had gone downhill overnight, and was having trouble breathing. As Caputo-Seidler's team worked to stabilize him, she was informed that a new patient was coughing up large amounts of blood and had been intubated and put on a ventilator. Her team ran to see the patient, whose oxygen levels were dangerously low, and took him to interventional radiology to determine the source of the bleeding. After bringing him back to the ICU, a nurse called to say the first patient was coding, so the team rushed back to perform CPR. They worked for a good hour trying to resuscitate him before the attending called the time of death. The patient's sister, who had been watching and begging him not to die, threw herself on top of the body, crying. "At this point I'm kind of choking back tears because again, I was already kind of emotional," Caputo-Seidler said. She was explaining to the residents about her father when they received a call that the other patient was bleeding, and they had to stabilize him again. By the time the necessary care for both patients had been provided it was early afternoon, and Caputo-Seidler went to the bathroom and cried. "I took about ten minutes, washed my face, and then we still had probably fifteen or so other patients that we hadn't seen yet, that we had to go round on," she said. "What's so hard is that often in the moment there's no time, there's no space for your own emotional response in these situations because there's the next patient who emerges and needs your attention and you just have to shut down whatever's going on."

When such emotions are not dealt with and processed, however, they can accumulate—with devastating consequences. When asked how first responders process grief, Jabr said, "I don't think they do." She often discusses *disenfranchised grief*—grief that's not openly acknowledged, socially validated, or publicly mourned—with the firefighters and paramedics she educates, and she found that one man was "just blown away" when the concept explained why he'd felt sad or upset over patient deaths—emotions he'd previously dismissed, telling himself he hadn't known the person. Other cases hit closer to home: Jabr recalled a firefighter-paramedic friend who'd responded to a call involving two police officers he knew who'd been killed. He left work early, and took the next couple of days to spend time with his family. Now, each year on the anniversary of their deaths, he pours out some beer to honor them. "Grief is grief, and it's going to look different for everybody," Jabr said. "If you're never able to open up and say, 'Hey, this bothers me, I just need to get it out,' it turns into something bigger than it would have been if you'd just gone through those emotions in the first place."

Kenneth Doka, a leading researcher in the field of grief and loss who coined the term *disenfranchised grief* in 1985, said that healthcare workers experiencing patient deaths would fall into the category of disenfranchised grief where a relationship isn't recognized. "I think there's still an attitude out there that healthcare workers should provide a distance," he said. "Healthcare workers, especially nurses' aides and things like that, often find their grief disenfranchised." Doka added that some institutions are better than others at recognizing and acknowledging the grief experienced by clinicians, while healthcare workers can also disenfranchise themselves for various reasons, such as the belief that becoming attached conflicts with their professional role. To better support their staff and prevent burnout, occupational stress, and turnover, health-care organizations "need to provide support, education, and sometimes ritual" to process patient deaths, he said.

Dizon said that writing about grief-laden experiences on his blog and on social media has been a "godsend" to processing his emotions. While he posts more for himself than for others, Dizon also benefits from colleagues who resonate with and respond to his words. "You realize that the experience, even though it's painful, is one that other people have also experienced," he said. "And then that sense of iso-lation goes away." For similar reasons, Dizon enjoys participating in Schwartz Rounds at his hospital—a program created by The Schwartz Center for Compassionate Healthcare that offers healthcare workers regularly scheduled times to discuss the social and emotional aspects of a patient's case with others in the field. Still, Dizon always finds himself disappointed by the low physician turnout. "It's a missed opportunity," he said. "So many of us suffer silently, and I think trying to go beyond that is still a challenge."

Caputo-Seidler, who'd like to see opt-out—rather than opt-in—counseling sessions for both medical students and faculty become more common, meets with a personal therapist outside of the university, and uses journaling as a tool for emotional release. "I'm somebody who by nature bottles things up," she said. "So I like journaling because that's something I can do by myself." Caputo-Seidler also teaches a humanities course for medical students, which she's found helpful for discussing the general challenges of the work, decompressing from her clinical experi-ences, and sharing coping mechanisms. She feels encouraged by medi-cal students and residents who embrace a cultural shift toward greater openness and emotional processing, but recognizes that it's slow going. "I think the culture is still very much, 'You keep your emotions to your-self,' and that's why we see such high rates of suicide and depression amongst physicians," Caputo-Seidler said. "Even if the patient doesn't die, you probably have to do something really hard, and have a really tough conversation, on a daily basis."

Making It Personal

After a young man died of a gunshot wound in his emergency room in 2018, Louis Profeta, a physician practicing in Indianapolis, picked up the patient's faded driver's license and held it in his large hands, pondering. Then, he opened his iPhone and went to Facebook. "He was about the same age as my kids," Profeta said. "A lot of times some of these people are friends with my kids, and I flipped on Facebook just to see who he was. And then I found myself looking at him a little differently." The experience later became the basis for Profeta's viral LinkedIn post, "I'll Look at Your Facebook Profile Before I Tell Your Mother You're Dead." In the article, Profeta expressed his anger at young patients for dying—and hurting their parents—and then assuaged it by discovering humanizing details on social media: "your smile, how it should be, the color of eyes when they are filled with life, your time on the beach, blowing out candles, Christmas at Grandma's; oh you have a Maltese, too." Still, he wrote the piece not to help physicians process their own grief, but rather, as a framework for parents to discuss the consequences of reckless behavior with their children. "That was the whole idea—to give parents the words to tell their kids that this is what love looks like," Profeta said.

Medical providers are often saddled with the horrendous task of telling family members that their loved one has died. They watch as parents, siblings, or children collapse in grief, wail in anguish, or react with anger. "You're kind of lucky that you don't have to see it," Profeta wrote in his piece. "Dad screaming your name over and over, mom pulling her hair out, curled up on the floor with her hand over her head as if she's trying to protect herself from unseen blows." Sharing information with patients about their worsening conditions or impending death is not much easier, and failing to do so effectively can harm both patients—leaving them confused about where they stand—and providers, who end up feeling guilty and frustrated. Yet while effective communication is essential to patient care, processing grief, and providing closure, many clinicians haven't received adequate training on how to handle such conversations.

Profeta, who's been an emergency physician for some twenty-five years, said that some of the most unimaginable situations have involved multiple family members who've been injured in a car crash or other traumatic accident. Once, he had to tell a young man that his infant had a brain injury, and his wife and little boy had both been killed. "Part of your soul dies," Profeta said. "It's the worst thing in the world." To balance out such tough days, he makes a concentrated effort to hone in on the more positive aspects of his work. "I come home from a busy day, and I've comforted some people, I've helped people feel better, and saved some people's lives," he said. "The key is to focus on that."

Numann said that she also struggled with delivering bad news to family members who'd been hospitalized following an accident. "They'll always ask, 'How's my husband? How's my son?'" she said. While Numann would occasionally delay bad news when a patient was highly unstable or suffering from amnesia, she'd otherwise "break it to them gently" by first discussing how bad the situation had been, then, by letting them know that everything had been done to help their loved one, but they hadn't survived. Numann would say if she believed the patient hadn't suffered, while employing softer terms such as "very bad head injury" rather than "decapitated" when asked for details. Once, a young patient with metastatic breast cancer was in the hospital with a broken hip when her father died on his way to visit her. Another woman was hospitalized with a serious illness when her husband suffered a lethal heart attack at home. Still, Numann—who credits the "feminization of medicine" with increasing acceptance of emotions in the field—was typically careful not to cry around patients, who could take it as a negative indicator of their condition; instead, she reserved her tears for funerals. Aside from the death of her sister, the only time Numann recalled crying at work was when a young man died in a motorcycle crash, and she went out to tell his mother. After Numann had explained organ donation—standard procedure at the time, but not something doctors typically do anymore—the mother thanked Numann, and said she wished she'd known that a year prior when her other son had died. "I can cry today thinking about it— how a mother can lose two sons," said Numann, her voice breaking.

Prior to death, bad news is often delivered directly to the patients themselves. News such as: Your tumor has progressed. This condition is now life-limiting. You are dying. Dizon—who developed his preferred methods of discussion from years of watching mentors and who always encourages students and residents to tag along for such conversations—said the first time he meets patients, he addresses their mortality directly. If he thinks he can control their cancer, or even cure it, he'll say he doesn't think they're dying. But he also assures them that if and when that changes, he'll let them know. "That is a very important statement, because it builds trust from the beginning," said Dizon, who will remind patients of the conversation if their condition progresses. Like most clinicians, Dizon is careful to use the words "death" and "dying" rather than softer euphemisms such as "not much longer to live" that are open to interpretation. And he avoids terms like "cancer patient" and "failed treatment" that he's learned from patients can communicate dehumanization or judgment. Instead, he'll frame patient care discussions around specific goals—whether he thinks an individual can make it to a highly-anticipated wedding, or to Christmas—and share his own feelings. "If I'm angry that the treatment didn't work, I'll say it's frustrating to me," he said.

When patients don't fully understand what their doctor is saying about their progressing condition or impending death, nurses will typically step in to answer questions and provide emotional support. "When someone hears that news, their mind goes off in many directions," Overcash said. "I don't know that they hear much after it." After a medical team leaves, Overcash often finds herself explaining things to patients, and "helping them to process, being empathetic." She answers questions, follows up with outpatient clients by phone, and provides ongoing support. "Some people feel that grief and anxiety every time they come to the cancer center," she said. "It doesn't go away." Overcash finds her ability to effectively engage in these conversations has improved with time, practice, and maturity. "As a professor, I don't know that we have any curriculum in preparing someone to speak to someone therapeutically," she said.

While doctors and nurses have traditionally had to figure out their own approach to delivering or expanding on bad news, medical training programs have been making a greater effort to prepare physicians for conversations around prognosis and end-of-life goals. Anthony Back, an oncologist and palliative care specialist, was shocked when, as a medical student, he witnessed an attending physician fail to inform a patient with life-threatening preleukemia how serious her condition had become. She died that night in the emergency room, and the following morning the doctor said, "Well, I guess she was just an old trout." Back felt terrible. "She had no chance to really understand what she was up against," Back said. "That was the beginning of my understanding of what all this meant."

Back, who is now an oncologist and professor of medicine at the University of Washington in Seattle, spent over a decade doing research on oncologist-patient communication—but still, he felt it wasn't enough. There were more than seventeen thousand oncologists practicing in the US, and even if they read his research, only those who'd participated would gain any practical experience. So instead of doing yet another study, Back and his colleagues founded VitalTalk, a nonprofit that trains clinicians to have hard conversations through role-plays with trained actors and by providing feedback. Since 2012, VitalTalk has trained nearly seven hundred clinician faculty around the country, and has reached some twenty-five thousand participants nationwide—with a focus on doctors, nurse practitioners and physician assistants. "A lot of data showed doctors are really not interested, and yet doctors are the ones who are the leverage point for decision making," Back said. "They have been the hold-up, so we really wanted to focus on providers."

Back said that delivering bad news poorly can not only traumatize patients, cause them to be uninformed when making decisions, and damage their trust in medical care, but it can also leave doctors feeling guilty. "When they're not really being honest, when they haven't really put things out there, I think it eats away at them," Back said. "And it's frustrating for them, because patients will come back with the same questions or the same issues over and over." Instead, VitalTalk teaches providers to learn to see emotion, sit with it, and respond to it—resulting in much more caring and effective communication. And for those who don't have time? "You can figure out how to use even a short piece of time in a beneficial way," Back said. "What doctors need to know is that by investing a small amount of time in doing a good job giving serious news, they will end up saving loads of time and trouble for themselves later."

Some residencies have begun to include more formal training around difficult conversations. Samuel Slavin, an internal medicine resident at Massachusetts General Hospital, said he was surprised to discover the utility of Ariadne Labs' four-page "Serious Illness Conversation Guide" that breaks conversations down into five steps and suggests phrasing for sharing a prognosis such as "I wish we were not in this situation," and "I'm worried that this may be as strong as you will feel." Despite the boilerplate structure and seemingly obvious turns of phrase, Slavin was impressed by its ability to serve both patients and providers. "I think the key, the core of it, is that it makes it personal," he said.

As the end of life approaches, conversations begin to revolve around final treatments, and whether to choose a full code (full resuscitation, including CPR), a limited code (which permits some interventions but not others) or a Do Not Resuscitate (DNR) order. Profeta, who experiences a death roughly every third shift he works, said that one of the most gratifying parts of his job is helping people to realize when a full code will not serve them. "A lot of these people have widely metastatic cancer, or end-stage kidney failure, and horrible illnesses, and the family sort of hasn't come to grips that this is the end," he said. "You go up there and pull them aside and say, 'Hey, don't do this.' You're able to talk them out of it, and just let them go peacefully." Profeta said that he encourages his younger colleagues to do the same; to have the courage to say, "Listen: If this was my father or mother, this is what I'd do."

In recent years, paramedics and EMTs have been placed in the relatively new position of having to determine the time of death themselves. Jabr, who as a paramedic was grateful to leave patients and their families at the hospital, said first responders—who've often received minimal training around death communication—can be somewhat resistant to this expectation, not realizing that it's preferable to repeatedly transferring a patient between various responders and hospital staff. "At that point, the person delivering the news is so disconnected from what actually happened on scene that the family member, whether they consciously realize it or not, is left with this empty, inconclusive feeling," said Jabr, who personally found the paramedics' ongoing presence at her mother's death, for the two hours up until they called it, incredibly comforting. "Really at the core of our avoidance is our discomfort with death, our discomfort with failure."

One benefit of having paramedics call deaths in the field, Jabr said, is that they can genuinely assure family members that they did all they could—particularly when they've had to begin CPR. "We understand that we can do everything right and the patient still dies, but the family does not," she said. Such closure can be essential to providers as well. After receiving repeated questions about the outcomes of several pediatric drownings, Jabr and two colleagues developed a process they called "integrated conclusion of care" that created objective case notes from the dispatcher's call through the patient's hospitalization and distributed them to the staff involved. While the program lacked the administrative support necessary to keep it running, it was popular for providing broad, inclusive, and often imperative information. "What it offered was closure not only for the field providers, but also for the dispatchers," Jabr said. "They're the ones who literally have to listen to the family members screaming because they found their loved one dead and try to get them to engage."

Closure was especially difficult for many clinicians to find during the COVID-19 pandemic, when patients—whether they had contracted the illness or not—were dying alone, without their loved ones present. Caputo-Seidler, who spent much of the pandemic alternating between the COVID unit and the non-COVID unit at her hospital, found that lack of closure was one of the hardest aspects of an increasingly stressful job. She recalled one critically ill, COVID-19-free man, who'd been transferred from a nursing home, where he'd already been isolated from his husband for months. Caputo-Seidler cared for him for several days, relaying his condition over the phone. When he took a turn for the worse, she brought his husband in under an emergency exception for end-of-life situations. She met him in the patient's room to discuss their plan, but because this was the first time the couple—who'd been together more than forty years—had been able to interact in weeks, she found herself standing back. "The patient was unresponsive, but his husband was talking to him, and hugging him, and brushing his hair," Caputo-Seidler said. Eventually, she let the husband know that the patient had hours left to live, and they decided against resuscitation. About a half-hour after Caputo-Seidler left the room, the patient died. "He basically got an hour to say goodbye because of COVID," said Caputo-Seidler, who found herself assuaging the husband's guilt over not being more present. "I think he really appreciated me saying, 'None of this was your fault, this was the pandemic and our rules preventing you from doing what I know you would have done for your husband.'"

The longer she's in medicine, the more Caputo-Seidler has realized the importance of carving out time for closure and other forms of emotional processing—both with patients and with staff. As faculty, she tries to spend at least a few minutes discussing patient deaths with students and residents, sharing whether she feels sad, or disappointed, or wishes she'd better anticipated the outcome. "Just trying to normalize some of those emotions," said Caputo-Seidler, who, in addition to the regular challenges of the job, has struggled with overwork and insomnia during the pandemic; the fear that she's being pushed so hard she could make a mistake. "We have to give terrible news—we have to tell people that they're dying, that their treatments aren't working, that there's nothing left to try. And trying to be distant about that, it's a lot more work than just openly admitting that this sucks, and I'm sorry."

"The Change Is So Slow"

Some clinicians feel that their responsibilities—and the difficult conversations required of them—extend far beyond their medical role, particularly when socioeconomic factors play a part in their patients' ongoing decline. While more than a third of graduating medical students intend to care primarily for underserved populations, those who do so often say their grief is compounded by their inability to address the impact of widespread health disparities on patients. Particularly for underrepresented minority clinicians who've chosen to serve their communities, grief over patients' chronic and terminal illnesses is inextricably linked to much larger issues of racial inequality, economic disparities, and social injustice.

As the daughter and granddaughter of Mexican migrant farmworkers in Oregon, Eva Galvez was inspired to become a doctor by witnessing the health challenges in her community and watching her grandmother struggle with poorly controlled diabetes, partly due to linguistic and cultural barriers. Now, Galvez—who's been working for some ten years as a family physician at the Virginia Garcia Memorial Health Center, a community health provider that serves a largely Latino population east of Portland—revels in the opportunity to serve patients that remind her of her own family in a setting that "feels like home."

Still, Galvez struggles with the challenges confronting her patients. "The skills I learned in medicine aren't necessarily the things that I can use if people are having difficulty with immigration or housing, or suffering from trauma," said Galvez, who would like to see more medical school training on managing social determinants of health. "They're problems that we may be able to fix, but it's going to take more than just doctors and it's going to take years." Galvez was particularly struck by the situation of Latinos when the COVID-19 pandemic hit. Her clinic was on the front lines, providing testing at centers, drive-thrus, and mobile clinics. When it became clear that Latinos—many of whom are essential workers—were twenty times more likely than other patients to have the virus, Galvez became even more of an advocate, pushing for more testing, improved mitigation measures, and more culturally appropriate educational tools for migrant farmworkers. Many were living in cramped conditions, afraid to speak up for fear of losing their jobs but also out of fear of deportation. The pandemic shone a light on health challenges that had long been in place. "COVID is a disparity," Galvez said. "But what about diabetes and renal disease? Those have been there all along."

In April 2020, Galvez lost her first patient to COVID-19. She had a close relationship with his Guatemalan family, and because his hospital care team didn't have much support for Spanish-speakers, his family and physicians called her about twice a day for a month until he died. "That was very, very difficult," said Galvez, who found herself, in addition to her regular duties, enmeshed in challenging conversations around his care. "If that had continued, I could see where I could have gotten burned out." Other times, Galvez finds herself deeply affected by patients' traumatic stories—particularly those close to her age, such as women who've been sexually assaulted or lost children when crossing the US-Mexico border.

Over the years, Galvez has developed methods of creating space for herself—stepping back from the news, and from work, so she can let go. She spends time with her husband and two children, connects with girlfriends, and goes for early morning walks or runs during which she says a prayer of gratitude. "There's even guilt sometimes in that because I can step away, and my patients can't," she said. "But I also think that if I don't give myself that space then I'm not going to be there for anybody."

The one time Galvez recalls losing control in front of a patient was a particularly challenging day—one similar to many. She'd skipped lunch. She hadn't had a restroom break. She'd seen multiple patients with complex social and emotional needs. And she was late. When she entered the room where a mother who'd been waiting with her child lashed out at her for taking so long, Galvez broke down crying. The mother, whom Galvez knew quite well, immediately apologized. Galvez said she was sorry; she'd just had a hard day. "We hugged, and I got things together, and we had the visit," Galvez said. "But that was I think the only time in my life where I completely let my guard down." Afterward, Galvez wrote a letter to herself to process her feelings, which she shared with her husband and sister, both physicians. In doing so, she realized she'd been feeling especially vulnerable because the person who'd been looking after her children for ten years had recently quit without warning. "That's why it's important for doctors to go into work being as well as they can," Galvez said. "Because if you're dealing with depression or anxiety or some kind of personal problem and then you go into an environment that's high stress, I could see where people could break."

Grief *on the* Front Lines

After obtaining her degree from the University of Minnesota Medical School, Mary Owen, a member of the Tlingit tribe in Alaska, also returned to serve her community and stayed for eleven years. "I knew about the inherent problems of mistrust," Owen said. "I knew about what it looks like not to be able to get to your appointment because you're prioritizing other family needs. I knew about physicians acting more powerful and less humble. So to have that knowledge was very empowering." Owen also drew on her understanding of the community's cultural history, interpersonal dynamics, and tribal politics to better connect with her patients.

Still, Owen found it challenging to witness the influence of poverty and other social inequities on her community's physical and mental health. "What's difficult for me isn't so much the grief from losing a patient, or grief from disagreeing with a patient over plans," Owen said. "It's more the grief that comes from not being able to fix things when people are suffering from depression because of real life circumstances." Owen would often prescribe medication for depression, only to find that patients didn't improve—because they were still living in the same house with black mold, or noise resulting from proximity to their neighbors and thin walls was causing stress, or some other condition remained unchanged. These stressors not only affected patients' mental health, but worsened their chronic physical conditions as well. And Owen bristled at simplistic solutions offered by others—such as the faculty member who told her, when she was a resident working in a primarily African-American population, that teaching people to use a pressure-cooker to prepare beans would resolve their dietary issues.

Owen, now the director of the Center of American Indian and Minority Health and an associate professor at the University of Minnesota Medical School, is hopeful that the greater awareness of racial inequities following the police killing of George Floyd in Minneapolis will make some difference. In the aftermath of the resulting protests, the University of Minnesota, which is one of the most successful recruiters of Native American medical students in the nation, began looking at increasing the number of curriculum hours spent on issues in Native American health. "This is the first time ever that everyone's saying, 'Yeah, we need this in our curriculum,'" Owen said, adding that medical schools also need to work harder to develop pipelines for minority students. When compared to the US Census total of 1.7 percent in population representation, a mere 0.2 percent of US medical school applicants in the 2018–2019 academic calendar identified themselves to be of Native American or Alaskan Native origins. Meanwhile, applicants of Hispanic, Latino, or Spanish origins were represented at 6.2 percent out of 18.5 percent total population, while a slight increase was displayed for applicants of Black or African-American origins, with 8.4 percent representation out of 13.4 percent total population.

Owen regularly confronts racial inequality in other forms—such as having to dress up to be taken seriously in the hospital, or being the only person of color in the room—and draws on her own patients' struggles to remain motivated. She recalled a recent Zoom meeting with all-white colleagues in which a lecture titled "Native Americans and Alcoholism" topped a list of class topics for redistribution—despite the fact that Native Americans and African-Americans are disproportionately affected by most diseases. "I felt the shame that I used to feel as a Native person in high school," she said. "My face was flushed. I felt just belittled and angry and sad and everything all at once." Owen, who uses exercise to work off some of her stress, also finds community activism invigorating, such as her involvement with the Equity Alliance to improve high school graduation rates for minority students. But sometimes, circumstances bring her down—such as when the pandemic reduced community involvement and she began to fear that the protests in the wake of George Floyd's death could be in vain. "Just the angst that the window will close, and nothing will happen," said Owen, who would like to see more underrepresented minority students in medicine, more people of color in positions of power, and curriculum that empowers students to address social determinants of health in their communities.

Rita Adeniran, an assistant clinical professor at Drexel University College of Nursing and Health Professions in Philadelphia, said she left clinical nursing because of the moral distress she experienced when she was unable to help patients suffering from health disparities in Philadelphia. The term *moral distress* was first defined by Andrew Jameton in his 1984 book *Nursing Practice: The Ethical Issues* to describe when a nurse "knows the right thing to do, but institutional constraints make it nearly impossible to pursue the right course of action." This definition has since been broadened to encompass other healthcare workers and other challenging situations, such as moral uncertainty, though some argue that the differences between these categories remain important to addressing the issue. "You want to do so much good but you cannot," Adeniran said. "Policies do not support you to do that, the resources are not there for you to do it, so you go home every day distressed."

Adeniran, who previously served as the director of diversity and inclusion for the University of Pennsylvania Health System and as a global nurse ambassador for the Hospital of the University of Pennsylvania, said she still encounters moral distress but on a "much bigger level." As an appraiser for the Magnet Recognition Program, Adeniran assesses hospitals that are hoping to achieve Magnet status for excellence in nursing and is often upset by their lack of diversity. "Some of it makes shivers run through my spine," she said. "Like the patient population you are serving is 30 percent underrepresented groups but your nursing staff is only comprised of 0.5 percent underrepresented groups." Adeniran is often informed that the hospital can't find qualified candidates, which is when she asks how far they've looked, and whether they have pipeline programs.

Adeniran, who grew up in a Nigerian village and was grateful for the opportunity to pursue a nursing career in the US, was inspired to become an advocate for diversity and inclusion from the beginning of her career. "I was flabbergasted to see the significant role that race and culture play in the US healthcare delivery and educational system," she said. "Everything in healthcare was modeled for the dominant culture. I wanted to be part of the solution." Over the years, she has had to learn to be "graciously assertive" when facing discrimination due to her dark skin and heavy accent, such as when a professor ignored her response to a question while recognizing the same answer when it was repeated by a native English-speaker.

Still, it can be draining. Adeniran, who has left jobs over her inability to make needed change, is often one of the few Black people at the table, and the only one with an accent. Sometimes, she'll come home after facing overt discrimination, or not receiving the outcome she's been hoping for, and "cry for days." As the wife of a Black man and the mother of three Black boys in their twenties who've suffered significant family trauma due to their race, her motivation is personal as well as professional. "The change is so slow," said Adeniran, who draws strength from her husband's initiative to start his own nondiscriminatory healthcare organization, as well as the generations of African-Americans who've suffered much longer. "I would love it to be faster, but it's happening."

Grief can take many forms: the anguish Adeniran experiences over an inability to make needed change; the clinicians who watch family members collapse over the loss of their loved ones; exposure to the slew of influences—only some of which are medical—that contribute to patients' ongoing decline and eventual death. Yet there are few avenues available to express the emotional fallout of these experiences. Some, such as Profeta and Dizon, turn to social media; others, like Caputo-Seidler, to journaling. Some make use of Schwartz Rounds, while others, such as Owen and Galvez, find hope in advocating for change. Acknowledging the impact of these experiences is the first step toward creating better structural support systems, improving medical curricula, and developing initiatives to confront the difficult conversations, racial and socioeconomic inequality, and other devastating aspects of working in healthcare.

3

Environmental Hazards

Violence is not power, but the absence of power.

—RALPH WALDO EMERSON

Whether they work in rural or urban environments, with underserved or privileged patients, doctors, nurses, and other healthcare workers always encounter significant environmental challenges. Not only do they suffer the grief and trauma of patient deaths—much of which goes unrecognized—but they are also repeatedly traumatized by exposure to disease, workplace violence, bullying by peers or supervisors, and other dangers—some of which are life-threatening. Like grief, many of these hazards remain disenfranchised in that they are poorly acknowledged, supported, or addressed by healthcare systems, which commonly seek easy fixes such as self-care and resiliency training. Yet these challenges require more direct action: healthcare workers have reported back injuries, chemical exposures, and infected needle sticks in addition to extreme stress, and have some of the highest rates of nonfatal occupational injuries and illnesses of any industry, according to the US Bureau of Labor Statistics (BLS).

Initially, the COVID-19 outbreak highlighted the hazards of working in healthcare—in part, due to widespread shortages of personal protective equipment—and boosted popular support. Americans cheered or banged pots and pans in windows to demonstrate solidarity during lockdowns, chalked encouraging illustrations on sidewalks outside hospitals, and delivered meals to frontline workers. Yet as the months wore on and these initiatives faded, many clinicians not working in critical care were furloughed or even lost their jobs, while the number of healthcare workers succumbing to the virus continued to rise. By September 2020, the Centers for Disease Control and Prevention (CDC) had tallied close to 700 healthcare worker deaths, while an independent analysis by *The Guardian* and Kaiser Health News counted hundreds more. The majority were people of color, revealing the racial and economic inequality inherent in healthcare settings: lower-paid healthcare staff working closely with patients such as nurses, nursing home employees, and support staff were much more likely than doctors to die from the virus. In addition to those who died, many others suffered through a frightening, and sometimes extended, illness.

For some, such as Julianne Viviano, an ICU nurse at a Level I trauma center in Brooklyn, one of the worst aspects of falling ill during the pandemic was the moral distress of being unable to help.

"Weighing Always on the Back of My Mind"

Early on in the pandemic, Viviano was working at her converted COVID-19 unit, when she suddenly came down with a fever of 104, fatigue, and general malaise. Fortunately, she didn't have any respiratory symptoms. "I just felt awful," she said. "I had already seen very young patients that had gotten critically ill, so I was very scared." Viviano, who lived alone with her German Shepherd, Apollo, had to reassure her parents in Syracuse and convince her mother not to drive down while she waited out the illness. After about five or six days, her fever began breaking during the day, but returning again at night. "It was frustrating because I wanted to be able to help," she said. "So there were a lot of mixed emotions during that time." Once she was seventy-two hours free from fever, per protocol,

Viviano returned to the ICU, where she was swabbed five days later. The test came out negative, but considering her exposure and the fact that testing was highly inconsistent at the time, she likely had COVID-19.

Viviano's patients were less fortunate. Her fourteen-bed unit housed the hospital's most critically ill, and of the hundreds that cycled through over the months, she only ever saw one, an elderly woman, recover. The others died—sometimes as many as five a day, sometimes within minutes of being transferred. At the height of the surge, for two to three weeks in April, nurses repurposed from other areas of the hospital began handling the postmortem care—cleaning and preparing the body for viewing or transport to the morgue—so that beds could be freed up more quickly, and "it was just like this revolving door." After work, Viviano would come home and cuddle with Apollo, have a glass of wine, or just shower and go straight to bed—the earlier the better, as she would hear ventilator alarms in her sleep. "For a long time you really can't process it," she said. "Because if you do, if you really sit down and think about it, you wouldn't be able to get up and go to work the next morning."

Another nurse at an Oklahoma nursing home, who asked not to be named for fear of repercussions, became terrified of endangering her two children following a COVID-19 outbreak at the facility. In May 2020, two patients who had tested positive were sent to the hospital, and she was furious when nobody informed the nursing staff until days later. She was tested, and her eleven-year-old son stayed with his grandmother, and her eight-year-old daughter with her dad, with whom she shared custody, while she waited for the results. "There were two weeks where I didn't even get to see my kids," she said. After taking some personal time off for other reasons, she was once again not informed there were positive cases in the facility; not long after her return, administrators formally announced dozens of positive cases and two deaths. "I don't mind taking care of COVID patients," she said. "But notifying your staff the minute you know that test is positive should be a no-brainer." Every time her children sneezed, she became anxious, and she found it hard to unwind in the evenings by chilling out and watching TV. Instead, she was constantly looking in their rooms and checking on them.

Even when there's not a global pandemic, clinicians are at risk for contracting serious illnesses such as HIV, Hepatitis B and C, and syphilis. The fear created by exposure can be highly anxiety-provoking and is an especially significant concern for those working in emergency rooms and ICUs where the risk of contagion is higher. Emergency physician Gregory Bledsoe was working as the lone doctor on a busy night shift when a patient came in who'd tried to kill himself by slitting his wrists. Bledsoe, who was exhausted and distracted from managing ten or fifteen other patients, eventually found time to stitch him up, and they got to chatting. Bledsoe had seen from the patient's record that he was a poorly compliant HIV carrier with high viral loads, so he was double-gloved, and taking all the usual precautions. But just as he was putting in the final stitches, Bledsoe felt a prick on one finger. "I looked down and could see a bead of blood underneath my glove," he said. "And so I finished the repair and ran to the sink and washed it off."

Bledsoe knew that a stick from a solid bore needle, rather than an injectable needle, was low risk, even with significant viral loads. But he was still worried. He was tested, in accordance with hospital protocol, and went on retroviral medication for a month—though it took hours for them to locate the right meds. "I was worried about the delay," said Bledose, who was rechecked at thirty days, and then again at six months, at which point he knew he was in the clear. He had to go home and tell his wife, who was also concerned. "It was weighing always on the back of my mind," he said.

For Rosalind Kaplan, an internist who probably had more than one needle stick during her residency at an urban Pennsylvania hospital in the late '80s, the consequences weren't immediately apparent. Kaplan had just finished residency and was married with a new baby when she had some abnormal liver function tests that failed to improve over time. Eventually she saw a GI doctor, who gave her an antibodies test for a newly isolated virus: Hepatitis C. Kaplan was positive. And since she hadn't used IV drugs or received a blood transfusion, she knew it had to be from work.

"I was a wreck," Kaplan said. "It was really harrowing." During her residency, she'd cared for people with what was then known as "non-A, non-B hepatitis" in the ICU, and many had died in horrific ways from liver failure and enlarged veins in the esophagus, or varices, that would bleed out. "You'd just see blood all over the walls and the ceiling," Kaplan said, adding that the way these patients were treated at the time was to insert a balloon device in their esophagus to tamponade the bleeding, and secure it by connecting it to a football helmet on their head. "So I started thinking, 'Oh my God, I'm going to have liver failure, I'm going to need a liver transplant, or I'm going to end up having an esophageal bleed like this and be like one of these patients in the ICU.'"

Because the condition was relatively new and there wasn't much information about it, Kaplan was also worried about passing it on to family members. She decided against breastfeeding her baby—Hepatitis C can't be transmitted through breast milk, but that wasn't clear at the time. Kaplan underwent multiple experimental treatments, the third of which finally cured her—eight years later, though it was longer before she could be confident she wasn't in remission. "For those eight years I was sort of plodding through things and being very tough on the outside, but I was really distraught," Kaplan said. She fought with her husband who, frustrated at being unable to fix things, would just try to say something positive. "There was nothing that could calm me down," she said. "I was really not consolable."

Despite the traumatic nature of the experience, Kaplan, who documented her journey in her book, *The Patient in the White Coat: My Odyssey from Health to Illness and Back,* found over time that there were some upsides. "It gave me a lot more perspective and compassion," she said. "I couldn't look at myself as distanced from people who were ill, and I think that actually probably made me a better doctor." Though her friends helped her through, Kaplan would have appreciated some peer support at the time—especially when having to advocate for herself, such as when her first round of treatment with interferon caused depression, and she had to demand that she be prescribed antidepressants before a second treatment ensued. Kaplan has since been able to provide such support for others, who sometimes call her in panic after sticking themselves with a needle or after being diagnosed with hepatitis. "You draw

strength from doing that," said Kaplan, who—like many medical trainees and new doctors—would have benefitted from institutional support
rather than being forced to rely solely on her own resources and efforts
at self-care. "If I had somebody I could fall back on it would have been
helpful," she said.

"Don't Turn Your Back"

For Basem Khishfe, peer support is what got him through one of the
most trying episodes of his life. On November 19, 2018, Khishfe was one
of two doctors working in the emergency department at Chicago's Mercy
Hospital & Medical Center when his colleague, Tamara O'Neal, left for
the day a few minutes late. Shortly after, a clerk ran inside, shouting, "He
shot her! He shot her!" They called a code silver—the code for an active
shooter—and Khishfe, along with the rest of the staff, ran and hid as the
gunman entered the hospital. Some ten minutes later, the police arrived.
They killed the shooter—O'Neal's ex-fiancé—but not before he'd also
opened fire on a police officer and a pharmacist. Khishfe showed the
police, who'd locked down the emergency department, his doctor's
ID and asked if he could check on O'Neal. He found her lying on the
ground in the parking lot, in a pool of blood. "I think she was already
dead by then," Khishfe said, "but we tried everything." He performed
CPR on his colleague before she was sent to the University of Chicago
Medical Center, and then went back inside to try to save the others. They
didn't survive.

"In that moment you're just numb, you're kind of in denial, you're
not believing that you're living," Khishfe said. He'd worked with O'Neal
for almost a year and a half, and they'd become friends. Hospital administrators gave Khishfe the week off, but he showed up the next day to connect with his peers, regardless. "It was much harder not to be there, and
not to be with the people that you went through this with," he said. "It
was just good for closure." While Khishfe felt some guilt over the fact that
O'Neal had left late, and wondered if there was anything he could have
done differently, he eventually accepted that it hadn't been his fault.

Instead, the experience solidified his anti-gun stance, which, as someone from war-torn Lebanon, was already strong. Still, the next gunshot victim he encountered "brought all that day back."

Workplace violence is rampant in the medical industry. For both healthcare and social assistance sectors, three-quarters of occurring nonfatal assaults require days away from work for recovery purposes, according to data collected by the US Bureau of Labor Statistics (BLS) in 2018. Alarmingly, these numbers have been rising steadily since 2011. Emergency departments that serve patients who've suffered trauma, families in distress, and people under the influence or who are mentally disturbed, among other disruptive circumstances, are especially impacted. Nearly half of emergency physicians have reported acts of assault by patients at work, according to a large national poll in 2018, while over 70 percent have been witnesses to an assault. Additionally, about 70 percent of emergency nurses have been hit or kicked on the job, according to the Emergency Nurses Association (ENA).

Bledsoe, who spent twenty years working in some fifteen emergency departments around the mid-Atlantic, northeastern, and southern US, in both rural and urban areas, said he's been punched, kicked, and spit on many dozens of times—typically by patients who had psychiatric issues or were intoxicated. Once, a mildly intoxicated patient in his mid-fifties punched him with a closed fist, very intentionally, right in the face—an experience that not only left a bruise, but shook him, causing him to become wary not to let patients between himself and the door. "It makes you very, very jittery going to work," Bledsoe said, adding that while hospitals typically have security, they're often too afraid of upsetting patients or the potential of a lawsuit to use it. As a result, emergency personnel can feel alone in facing constant verbal and physical abuse, with no one to back them up. "It's basically the customer-is-always-right mentality applied to a very violent, unstable environment," Bledsoe said. Meanwhile, calling security can also backfire—on occasion, armed security personnel have shot and killed patients, and even staff. And racial profiling is a serious concern: one 2018 study found that security standby requests were called more than twice as often for Black patients in hospitals than their white counterparts, which could also induce some moral distress in healthcare workers when choosing whether or not to call.

At his current and previous positions in Arkansas, where he is also the state's surgeon general, Bledsoe said he's felt supported by hospital administration—partly because the CEO at his last hospital was a cardiologist with clinical experience. "There's a reason why we're hemorrhaging talent from [emergency medicine]," said Bledsoe, who would like to see more hospital leadership with clinical acumen in addition to business talent. "It would be great if the broader public, and then also the people who are making decisions for staffing and running hospitals, had a better understanding of the pressures on emergency personnel—physicians and nurses in particular—and listened to them," he said.

When encountering problems, healthcare administrators often seek outside analysts for help. After executives repeatedly asked the Advisory Board, which is headquartered in New York and consults with healthcare organizations in more than fifty countries, how to help staff become more resilient, its Nursing Executive Center published a 2018 paper, "Rebuild the Foundation for a Resilient Workforce." The paper drew on Maslow's hierarchy of needs, which states that unless people's basic physical needs for safety and survival have been met, addressing their psychological needs or desire for self-fulfillment is premature. Based on input from frontline nurses, healthcare leaders, and resilience experts, it identified four "foundational cracks"—the first of which was workplace violence and threats to point-of-care safety. "No one was really looking at what's at the base of the pyramid, which are what we consider those foundational needs," said Katherine Virkstis, a managing director and senior research partner at the Advisory Board. "If you don't have those, then it doesn't matter how much you put at the top, it will all crumble in on itself." The other three "foundational cracks" included moral distress resulting from institutional restrictions on delivery of care; lack of opportunity to recover from traumatic experiences; and changes in care delivery processes that left nurses feeling more isolated.

Workplace violence in healthcare isn't new. Mary Bennett, who is now retired but spent twenty-five years as a nurse at Parkland Memorial

Hospital in Dallas, recalled an incident in the '90s when a prisoner who'd been brought into the emergency room had managed to get a gun away from the guard accompanying him and was trying to shoot off his shackles. "He was going through the halls shooting this gun, and people were running," she said. Bennett and another nurse hurried into a room, passing an elderly lady with a broken ankle in the hall who was distressed and wanted to know what was happening, and wedged a gurney up against the door. "That was very frightening, just the scene of all the people, nurses and doctors, just running," Bennett said. She worried about the woman with the broken ankle and other patients left outside. Fortunately, nobody was injured in the incident—or in the two other active shootings at the hospital during her time there.

However, workplace violence has become more commonplace in recent years, costing US hospitals an estimated $2.7 billion in both proactive and reactive responses, according to a 2016 Milliman Research Report for the American Hospital Association. Data from the BLS show that nonfatal assaults in the healthcare and social assistance industry leading to days away from work increased 86 percent from 2011 to 2018, compared to 58 percent in other industries.

Meanwhile, BLS figures fail to account for verbal and physical assaults that do not result in time away from work–which are most of them, according to the previously mentioned 2018 poll of emergency physicians. They also exclude assaults that aren't reported, which are once again the majority. A study of about 450 employees across seven US hospitals, published in the journal *Workplace Health and Safety* in 2015, discovered 77 percent of violent incidents went unreported in any manner, while even fewer were logged in the hospital's electronic system. Contributing factors toward the failure to report include time-consuming reporting procedures, the normalized perception that such incidents are simply part of the job, and even fear of reprisal. Some nurses have been warned against alerting the authorities, with the looming threat of being fired for seeking legal reparations.

Suzie Couch, an operating room nurse at a hospital in the St. Louis area of Missouri, spent most of her more than twenty-year career in obstetrics, though she has also worked in orthopedics, corrections, education, and administration. In that time she's had to hold down patients who were violently flailing while waking up from anesthesia, and talk down anxious and verbally abusive visitors. During her ten months as a high-risk OB manager for a Missouri Medicaid vendor, Couch would follow up with patients who were drug users, had high blood pressure, were previously high-risk diabetics, or had other complications. Sometimes, she had to visit housing projects where she felt unsafe, and because company policy prevented her from carrying a weapon while on duty, she would grasp "nursing instruments" in her pocket, such as a big pair of bandage scissors. "It's what you have to do to get through," she said.

As she approaches her fifties, Couch has found that despite her sturdy, nearly six-foot frame, the strain of lifting heavy patients, staff shortages, and extensive charting requirements can become wearing. Still, she loves being a nurse, especially when she's able to empower patients who've been railroaded by the system in the past to take an active role in their healthcare. To stay positive, she works out on a Peloton spin bike, takes RV trips with her wife, and recites a "nursing mantra" paraphrased from Mahatma Gandhi: "Sometimes you find yourself by losing yourself in the service of others."

Unfortunately, that service isn't always appreciated. Couch—who attributes the growth in workplace violence to an increase in chronic health conditions, financial stress, and a litigious culture—has regularly had patients' family members scream profanities at her and threaten to sue, assault, or even shoot her. "I learned early on, don't turn your back," said Couch, who draws on skills honed from growing up with a bipolar mother to recognize nonverbal cues. Often, she said, nurses become so task oriented that they fail to notice the danger. In a recent incident at her current hospital, a patient body-slammed two nurses—one into the floor, and another into the wall.

The Advisory Board recommends that organizations address workplace violence by gathering data to determine the magnitude and nature of the problem; clearly defining acceptable verbal and physical behavior for patients and visitors and enabling staff to hold them accountable; and empowering staff to advocate for their safety by encouraging a culture of reporting. Their paper offers specific practices, such as a simple tool to assess potential behavioral escalation and take predetermined actions to intervene, as well as reducing response time for security personnel. "You need to actually shine a light on what does the workplace violence look like within your own organization," Virkstis said. "And it needs to include things like verbal abuse and intended assault where no injury occurred, because those are the things that are greatly underreported." She added that sometimes administrators' failure to take action comes from the fact that they simply aren't aware of the scope of the problem. In one such situation, she recalled that a nursing executive advocating for change had submitted daily reports for about two weeks to the C-suite, after which they were willing to invest in solutions.

In addition to patients and visitors, Bledsoe would like to see administrators and supervisors develop a greater awareness of how their behavior affects healthcare workers who are already grappling with extremely stressful jobs. He tries to offer positive feedback—something he rarely received early on in his career—and advises hospital leaders and managers to do the same. When asked what he'd say to healthcare workers who are struggling, Bledsoe replied: "You're doing an incredible service for the community. You're doing amazing work in a low-resource and high-stress environment and you are one of the important cogs in the machine of the community that keeps everything going. And if people aren't telling you that, that's on them, that's not on you. You matter and you need to realize that."

"Just Lashing Out"

Doctors, nurses, techs, and other hospital staff not only receive minimal positive feedback, but they're also demeaned, criticized, and even bullied. These negative experiences—and their invisibility—are likely connected to the larger refusal to acknowledge healthcare workers' grief, distress, and other very human needs and emotions. Such detrimental behavior often becomes ingrained in medical and nursing school, when students are commonly hazed and harassed by superiors, leading to the adoption of similar attitudes. Mikkael Sekeres recalled his first clinical rotation as a medical student in surgery—something he was seriously considering as a career. "I liked the combination of intellectualism and also using your hands, but was steered away from it because of how med students were treated," Sekeres said. "It was physical abuse; it was emotional abuse." The surgical staff at his Philadelphia hospital took a competitive, hierarchal, and almost militaristic approach, labeling certain students as "strong" and others as "weak" while taking pride in ignoring basic biological needs, such as food and sleep. Sekeres started work at 5 a.m. and stayed for twelve to fifteen hours; if anyone asked the chief resident what time they'd round out, the resident would purposefully add on an hour. Once, a cardiothoracic surgeon invited Sekeres to scrub in and, during the surgery, asked him to hold a patient's heart. "I held it as if it were Faberge, like it was the most delicate, fragile thing on the face of the earth," Sekeres said. "And he just started shouting at me. It was like a rite of passage." The surgeon accused Sekeres of almost tearing the patient's heart out, and threw him out of the operating room.

Operating rooms are notorious for being competitive, aggressive, and often hostile environments—partly because of the high status accorded to surgeons, the minimal room for error, and the elevated stakes: the cost expenditure in an operating room (OR) equates to roughly $40 per minute, according to data from California hospitals in a 2014 *JAMA* study. A strict hierarchy is typically observed, with the surgeon at the top, followed by their assistant—a registered nurse first assistant (RNFA), physician assistant, or surgical assistant—the circulating nurse; and then the scrub tech, who prepares, sterilizes, and hands instruments to the surgeon, among other duties. One scrub tech, who's spent sixteen years working in three US states and who asked not to be identified for fear of backlash, said she routinely felt underappreciated and burned out. Once, after stepping in to assist on an emergency heart operation that saved the patient's life, the heart team's nurse coordinator, who'd repeatedly told her that scrub techs weren't allowed on the heart team, arrived and told her to "get out." Later, this nurse coordinator acknowledged that the scrub tech had done a good job—but then reminded her that she wasn't permitted on the team. "You can only hear 'you're just a tech' for so long before you start believing it," the scrub tech said.

Nick Angelis, who's spent some ten years working as an agency nurse and nurse anesthetist in large hospitals and small surgery centers in Florida and Ohio, has seen surgeons hurl instruments across the OR more than once, narrowly missing a nurse. "That's the most dangerous one, because of course there's a lot of risk of contamination—everything's sharp and bloody," he said. "And that would be tolerated depending on how much money the surgeon brought in." Male surgeons are infamously insufferable in this manner, exemplifying what Joan Cassell, author of *The Woman in the Surgeon's Body*, called the "'Iron Surgeon'—powerful, invulnerable, untiring." Angelis found that while bullying in the OR often took the form of direct physical or verbal abuse, from nurse to nurse it was more passive-aggressive; often, the nurse targeted was one of the most competent. "A lot of what I've done in my career is go into toxic environments sort of like a substitute, because they couldn't find people who were willing to suffer that long-term, and see if I could change the culture and make it into a happier place," he said. Angelis, who alternates between goofy, engaging, and confrontationally joking, believes he tolerates bullying better than most due to his "weird personality" and individualistic nature.

Bullying has long been recognized as a problem in nursing. A 1986 article by Judith Meissner in the journal *Nursing* coined the phrase "nurses eat their young," and more than three decades later, it's still common vernacular. Cheryl Dellasega, an expert on relational aggression and author of *Toxic Nursing: Managing Bullying, Bad Attitudes, and Total Turmoil*, said the phrase is somewhat outdated, as these days there are plenty of second-career nurses, while other factors can also make one a target. Dellasega—now a professor of humanities at Penn State College of Medicine, as well as a professor of women's studies—was a nurse practitioner for most of her clinical career and has been the recipient of, witnessed, and may even have given the impression of bullying. "It has an impact on everybody involved," said Dellasega, who attributes its prevalence to the fact that nursing is a female-dominated profession and women have historically learned to express conflict psychologically, as well as the long hours and stress of the work. Early on in her career, Dellasega was taken under the wing of a more experienced nurse in the ICU who would "put the other nurses on the floor down and kind of criticize and harass them." She's seen nurses belittle others in front of patients or doctors and engage in harmful gossip, much of which has now been taken online. Nurses regularly contact her to share the resulting strain on their mental and physical health and to report that they've had to move floors, leave jobs, or quit the profession altogether. "With nurses, if your performance is criticized, that really gets to the heart of how you feel about yourself," Dellasega said. "It has a devastating effect on job turnover and burnout."

Renee Thompson, who's worked as a bedside nurse, in home care, as a frontline unit manager, in education, and in corporate, has experienced or witnessed bullying at all levels of the profession. As a new nurse, her preceptor—who was supposed to be training her—ignored her, refused to help her, and made her feel stupid for asking questions. "I was petrified that I was going to make a mistake," Thompson said. "It made me second-guess whether nursing was the right career." Eventually, Thompson's manager gave her a different preceptor and things improved. But after years of watching nurses engage in badmouthing, verbal aggression toward each other, and even actions harmful to patients—such as withholding essential information from other nurses—she decided to do something about it. About ten years ago, Thompson began working as a speaker, which eventually turned into a business: the Healthy Workforce Institute.

More than 180 hospitals around the country have since brought Thompson in to do year-long interventions; following one recent program in an operating room, she said that the director reported that employee engagement scores rose from 50 to 91 percent. Thompson begins with a survey that allows staff to discreetly identify problems and addresses the issues directly with them. After that, she implements a series of steps, including setting behavioral expectations and working with Human Resources to hold people accountable, as well as incorporating those expectations into performance reviews and one-on-ones.

Such policies can be particularly challenging to enforce during events such as the COVID-19 pandemic, when Thompson experienced a significant uptick in demand for her services. "People are so burned out, they're so stressed, that they're just lashing out at each other as a way to relieve that stress," she said. One nursing leader told Thompson she'd called a subordinate into her office after she went off on another staff member in front of a patient. But when the nurse removed her mask to reveal the way her face had been swollen and bruised by the PPE, the manager felt unable to reprimand her. Even when there isn't a pandemic, bullying and other aggressive behaviors are likely exacerbated by an inability to process the grief and trauma inherent to the medical profession. Similar to the manner in which child bullies often come from violent homes, clinicians can't help but be affected by their environments. Still, recognizing this impact doesn't negate the necessity to put a stop to bad behavior. "You can show empathy and care and compassion, but you have to address it," said Thompson, adding that doctors, managers, and staff with seniority must also be held responsible. "I would love to see more commitment at the executive level to address destructive behaviors independent of who's behaving in a destructive manner," she said.

Many doctors, nurses, and other healthcare staff are afraid to report their concerns to leadership, and those who do often find them dismissed outright. Sekeres, a physician at the Cleveland Clinic's department of hematology and oncology and a professor of medicine at Case Western Reserve University, said he chose an alternate specialty due to surgery's general culture of competition, almost constant hazing, and lack of interest in life outside of medicine. He completed a residency in internal medicine followed by a fellowship in hematology/oncology—where he also encountered "a lack of sensitivity that bordered on bullying." Sekeres had cared for people with cancer before, but this was the first time he and his colleagues had faced a patient population in which a large percentage would die. "I looked around at my fellowship class and saw that people were becoming clinically depressed," Sekeres said. His classmates were losing weight and becoming withdrawn; once, one of them sat beneath his desk and refused to engage. Yet when Sekeres raised his concerns with the fellowship head, he was told that everything was fine. He and the others embraced negative coping mechanisms, playing mean practical jokes on each other such as calling in fake consults to create unnecessary work. "It was a dysfunctional reaction to not being supported by anybody else," Sekeres said. "We wound up essentially bullying each other, emulating the treatment we were receiving from our supervisors." Now, Sekeres tries to lead by example when working with medical students, whose admissions essays reveal such hope and altruism. "If we're truly going to be empathic providers to our patients, we can't be hurting more than our patients," he said.

Alan Rosenstein, a practicing internist in San Francisco and a healthcare management consultant, was inspired to study disruptive physician behavior when working as a medical director and vice president at VHA West Coast, a group purchasing organization (GPO) servicing some two thousand member hospitals around the country. Because hospitals regularly cited disruptive physicians as being among their top ten issues, Rosenstein, who had personally witnessed "yelling and screaming and just derogatory, rude, demeaning behaviors," began conducting surveys to determine their impact.

The results were concerning. Not only did disruptive physician behavior reduce nurse satisfaction and retention, but it also had a negative impact on patient care. "People get so frustrated with others that they don't talk to them, they withhold information, they can't focus on what they're doing, they're afraid to ask them if they have a question," Rosenstein said. "And that's when bad things happen." In 2008, *The Joint Commission Journal of Quality and Patient Safety* published one survey consisting of more than 4,500 doctors, nurses, and other healthcare workers at over 100 hospitals. Alarmingly, this survey discovered 77 percent identified as witnesses to disruptive behavior in physicians, 65 percent as witnesses in nurses, and a collective 67 percent believed that such unruly behavior was correlated to adverse patient events. Meanwhile, there have been anecdotal accounts of patients feeling bullied by harried doctors.

Despite the prevalence of such behavior, Rosenstein said that "people tend to look the other way." To combat disruptive behavior, he said, healthcare organizations must develop effective policies and procedures and be willing to follow through, even when the offender is a prominent physician who is a good clinical provider. Rosenstein, who acknowledged that administrators can also behave badly, advised management to better support physicians by providing coaching, by establishing forums such as town-hall meetings in which physicians can vent their concerns and be heard, and by soliciting physician input on administrative decisions. "The leadership and the organizational culture are crucial background issues," he said.

Angelis, who would like to see better mental health support for healthcare professionals as well as bullying policies that are "led by wisdom and the nuance of the situation," became increasingly interested in mental health and opened his own healthcare organization, Alleviant Health Centers of Akron, in 2019. A year later, his ten-employee operation was providing ketamine infusions, transcranial magnetic stimulation, counseling, and other services to the general public to deal with depression, neuropathic pain, post-traumatic stress disorder (PTSD), and other mental health disorders.

Angelis made the transition after suffering some personal trauma—a bad divorce, in addition to the ongoing workplace bullying—and watching others struggle through tough times. He connected with two other nurse anesthetists who'd responded to a student's post on Facebook asking for help because "he was being bullied so badly," and in 2012, the three of them launched Florida-based BEHAVE Wellness, which helps to train corporations and individuals in eliminating bullying, promoting wellness, and advocating for targets—particularly nursing students, who often don't speak up for fear that their evaluations could suffer. As an administrator, Angelis tries to practice what he preaches, giving employees time off for important occasions and asking them what other support they need. "If organizations can find the superstars and make sure that they're happy and filled, they'll actually make a lot more financial gain than if they ask, 'How can we just squeeze every dollar out of them?'" Angelis said.

Trauma, Burnout, and Distress

Traumatic stress cuts to the heart of life, interfering with one's capacity to love, create, and work.

—SHAILI JAIN

Five years before COVID-19 hit her unit in Brooklyn, Julianne Viviano, the critical care nurse who'd likely contracted the virus, was a few months into her first position in a Syracuse cardiovascular ICU when her husband was badly injured in a military convoy crash. He spent five days in a neurological ICU before the family decided to withdraw life support, and when Viviano returned to work after a two-month leave, she found the environment could be triggering. "I was feeling myself getting very burnt out emotionally, being in a similar setting," Viviano said. "I had a very hard time separating myself from the families just because I had so recently been in their position." Viviano ended up transferring into a post-anesthesia care unit in the same hospital and didn't return to critical care until she moved to Brooklyn in early 2017. Over the next several years, she began her master's degree in nursing education and began training new hires.

Then the pandemic hit New York City, and Viviano's COVID-19 patient load began to increase exponentially. "There was so much death," she said. "Every day was awful, and you knew that every single day after that was going to be worse." She spoke weekly with the therapist she'd had since her husband died, who she said told her: "We're not going to be able to unpack any of this until it's over, because when you keep getting retraumatized every single day you're in survival mode." Viviano was working four to five shifts of more than twelve hours a week until a large group of travel nurses arrived to help, and she could go back down to three. She spent her free time sleeping, maintaining her athletic frame by taking her dog Apollo out for a run, and Facetiming with friends and family.

Trauma, burnout, and other forms of distress are common among doctors, nurses, paramedics, respiratory therapists, and other healthcare workers. And while each has specific definitions and parameters, they often overlap. The American Medical Association defines burnout, which affects more than 40 percent of physicians, as "a long-term stress reaction characterized by depersonalization" that can include emotional exhaustion, cynical or negative attitudes toward patients, reduced empathy, and a feeling of decreased personal achievement. The American Psychological Association, meanwhile, defines trauma as "any disturbing experience that results in significant fear, helplessness, dissociation, confusion, or other disruptive feelings intense enough to have a long-lasting negative effect on a person's attitudes, behavior, and other aspects of functioning." Post-traumatic stress disorder (PTSD), which is listed in the Diagnostic and Statistical Manual of Mental Disorders (DSM), has the most specific diagnostic criteria, including exposure to actual or threatened death, serious injury, or sexual violence; intrusion symptoms such as flashbacks or nightmares; avoidance of stimuli related to the trauma; negative changes in mood and cognition; and heightened arousal and reactivity, among others.

Meredith Mealer, an associate professor of medicine at the University of Colorado Anschutz Medical Campus who studies burnout and PTSD among nurses, said that much of what clinicians report as burnout is actually "a lumped category of psychological distress" that can include compassion fatigue, moral distress, anxiety, depression, PTSD, and other forms. "Burnout as a concept is sort of this catch-all syndrome," she said, pointing out that survey instruments developed for any one of these concepts will often incorporate symptoms of PTSD, while PTSD remains the most rigorous diagnosis. "The main reason why I chose the topic of burnout and PTSD in nursing is because I was seeing a lot of my colleague nurses leave the bedside," said Mealer, who was herself a critical care nurse for many years. "They would tell me things like, 'I'm having nightmares,' or 'I'm just anxious all the time.' So that kind of prompted me to look into the symptoms nurses were experiencing." In a 2012 study published by the *International Journal of Nursing Studies*, Mealer found that close to 21 percent of ICU nurses met the full criteria for PTSD, while up to 80 percent exhibited at least one indication of burnout.

For Viviano, it wasn't until mid-July, after the unit had been terminal-cleaned and returned to its previous state, that the trauma really hit her. While grateful to no longer be immersed in constant death, Viviano missed the manner in which everyone had come together during the crisis. She was frustrated that the limited staff had been put on an overtime and hiring freeze, and that the travel nurses had been sent away. "We were all feeling afraid of a second surge," she said. By the end of July, Viviano wasn't sleeping well. The day before her shift, she was experiencing extreme anxiety, and by evening she was throwing up. Viviano took a leave of absence, and then resigned at the end of August. "It was not sustainable for me, and I knew that," she said. Still, Viviano—who embarked on a cross-country road trip with her new boyfriend, the first travel nurse she'd met during the pandemic—expected to return to nursing and finish her master's. "I think I will go back to critical care after taking a little breather," she said.

Multiplying the Stress

While working in an ICU at the epicenter of a global pandemic is uncommonly challenging, the crippling anxiety that Viviano experienced as a result of her job is far from unusual. Mary Buffington had her first panic attack during her final semester of nursing school in West Virginia, when she was overwhelmed with information and a fear of failure and "just rocking and crying hysterically." After graduation Buffington held various positions, changing jobs whenever she began to feel burned out, until she hit "intense burnout" in 2014 when working at a high-volume outpatient cancer clinic in California. The clinic was short-staffed, with multiple nurses leaving within a year, and Buffington rarely had time to eat lunch. She had an inordinately high volume of patients—sometimes nine at a time, undergoing complicated and potentially dangerous chemotherapy regimens—regularly clocked out hours later than scheduled, and commuted an hour each way in Bay Area traffic. "I was having panic attacks at least once a week, I was having to take anti-anxiety medicine to go to sleep every night, and I stopped actually listening to myself," Buffington said. "I paid no attention to things outside my work because my work had bled over my whole entire life." Eventually Buffington hit rock bottom—and even after leaving to take three per diem positions with more flexibility, she still experienced aftershocks. "I was always waiting for a doctor to be verbally abusive, to be expected to do more than I really had the energy to do," she said. "I was in this protective, defensive space all the time."

Buffington found it ironic that her worst experience of burnout occurred in California—the only state that mandates nurse-patient ratios in hospitals—but those ratios, which limit a nurse to five patients, didn't apply to outpatient clinics such as the one where Buffington worked. Meanwhile, California nurses have had to fight to keep that ratio intact: During the pandemic, many protested when Governor Gavin Newsom waived enforcement of nurse-patient ratios for three months and gave hospitals the option to apply for an extension. Jorge Rosales, a nurse on a medical surgical/telemetry unit at an urban hospital in northern California, said increasing ratios would strain already overwhelmed nurses and put patients at risk. "A nurse's regular work day involves stressed-out, anxious patients crying in pain, psych patients who can get aggressive and violent, management nitpicking our charting or other details, and stressed-out doctors projecting their own stress," Rosales said. "I deal with four to five patients a day, so to have six to eight as in other [US] states not only creates an unsafe situation with increased risk of mistakes or delay to care, but also multiplies the stress."

Many healthcare organizations are stretching their nurses thin due to a national nursing shortage. This shortage is expected to worsen as Baby Boomers age, heightening patient loads at the same time that many practicing nurses retire: the average age of registered nurses is 51, according to a National Nursing Workforce Survey from 2017. While the Bureau of Labor Statistics has estimated approximately 200,000 new nurses will be required annually through 2026, the same nursing survey found that the number of active registered nursing licenses had only increased by 261,275 within two years, translating to a shortage of roughly 140,000. In addition, more than 60,000 qualified applicants are turned away from nursing schools every year due to a lack of faculty and clinical training sites, according to the American Association of Colleges of Nursing (AACN).

Simultaneously, the US is facing a looming doctor shortage, with a predicted deficit of 54,100 to 139,000 primary and specialty care physicians by 2023. If access improves for underserved populations, these scarcity numbers can be anticipated to more than double, according to the Association of American Medical Colleges (AAMC). Contributing factors include population growth and aging, as well as a workforce in which two out of five active physicians will reach retirement age in the next decade. Meanwhile, supply is not increasing at the same pace as demand, in part because Congress placed a cap on the number of residency positions funded by Medicare in 1997—and hasn't changed it since. While the House and Senate are considering the implementation of new legislation, which should add at least 15,000 residency slots over five years, those additional doctors would only meet a suboptimal quarter of the nation's healthcare needs.

One specialty that has already been hit hard is urology—which treats prostate, testicular and bladder cancer, among other illnesses—with the American Urological Association attributing a lack of workforce diversity, poor rural access, and physician burnout to existing shortages. Fifty-four percent of urologists feel burned out—the highest rate of any specialty, according to the Medscape National Physician Burnout, Depression and Suicide Report 2020. These figures updated during the COVID-19 pandemic, with urology at 49 percent while concurrently outpaced by infectious diseases, rheumatology, and critical care.

Ilene Wong Gregorio, a urologist in southeastern Pennsylvania, said that four urologists in her geographical area had departed within three years—due to disability, death, early retirement, and a decision to stop practicing. Since then, she said, the remaining three have performed the work of seven people. "Our volumes are incredibly high," she said. "There's also the increased burden of the electronic medical records. That's how we spend most of our day now, just clicking away at the computer." An excess of bureaucratic tasks was the top reason for burnout listed on the Medscape report, followed by "spending too many hours at work" and a lack of respect from administrators, employees, or staff. In addition, the computerization of practice is a chief complaint, with many doctors expressing strong displeasure in the number of hours spent on non-impactful activities such as extensive charting, entering billing details, and other obligations demanded by the electronic health record.

Wong Gregorio said her practice is more challenging than some because she works at three different hospitals in addition to her office, meaning that there's no continuity of patient care and a lot of time is spent signing in and out. She feels bogged down by the patient load, drained by financial negotiations between patients, specialists, and insurance companies, and wonders whether her skills are well spent on quality-of-life conversations about urine incontinence and other issues that could easily be handled by a physician's assistant. "Sometimes I wonder whether I would be better off to humanity if I were doing something different," she said. "There are just some days where I feel very toxic, where I'm irritable, and it reflects in my interactions with most of my patients and my staff and it's not my normal demeanor." Wong Gregorio, a typically down-to-earth woman who's struggled with depression since college and sees a therapist when she can, has also found that the culture of medicine is "not very kind to the idea of being human and having weaknesses." She's found ways to combat burnout and depression—including getting massages, giving herself permission to watch or read something mindless, and writing: in recent years, she's published two young adult novels. Still, the mother of two said that the recent hiring of two new associates contributed most to her quality of life and wellness. "There's nothing more stressful than wanting to be home with your kids and not being able to," Wong Gregorio said.

Karen Kaufman, an obstetrician and gynecologist who said she felt burned out by the end of her residency in 2001, spent about fourteen years at a private practice in Colorado, where she was initially on call every fourth night for 36 hours. She continued on this schedule through her first pregnancy—up until the minute she went into labor—and was increasingly drained by the patient load and lack of personalized care. She was seeing twenty to thirty patients a day, for no more than fifteen minutes each—the maximum time that insurance would cover, unless it was a new patient—and was able to learn nothing about their psychosocial life, what they were eating, or whether they were exercising. "You kind of become a machine," she said. "It just became so unsatisfying." The demanding schedule took a toll on Kaufman's lithe physique, and she eventually gave up obstetrics to improve her sleep and stress levels. And while she found she could spend slightly more time with patients, she was still frustrated by insurance companies that refused to cover certain tests, such as ultrasounds for women whose mammograms showed dense breasts—a risk factor for breast cancer, but also a condition that could obscure its presence. She was working with a lot of perimenopausal and menopausal women, and became interested in integrative medicine as a way to provide more holistic health. In 2015, she left the practice group, and a year later opened up her own office, where she now spends forty-five minutes with each patient and follows up with personalized care. While demanding, she finds this approach "incredibly satisfying" because patient outcomes are far superior. She's also able to spend more time with her two teenaged children, feels more adequately reimbursed because she's not relying on insurance, and can better prioritize her sleep and self-care.

Female physicians have regularly reported more burnout than their male counterparts, a finding that has been attributed to disproportionate domestic duties and greater work-related stressors, including sexual harassment, lack of equal pay, and fewer promotions to leadership positions. Meanwhile, a handful of studies on race and burnout suggest minority groups are less likely to report burnout—findings that could stem from greater resilience, stigma that limits disclosure, or other factors; researchers say further study is required. Damon Tweedy, an associate professor of psychiatry and behavioral sciences at Duke University School of Medicine and author of *Black Man in a White Coat: A Doctor's Reflections on Race and Medicine,* said race added an extra dimension to the stressors of medical school—whether that was racist remarks made by professors, such as the one who asked him if he was in the classroom to fix the lights; a higher patient load because as a Black student doctor he was assigned most of the Black patients; or the extra pressure caused by the sense that "your success or failure isn't just your own, it somehow represents those who've paved the way for you and who will come after you." As Tweedy has advanced in his career, he's much less concerned about being judged based on race, but as one of the few Black faculty, he's often saddled with additional, unpaid "Black responsibilities" such as various committees targeted toward minorities. "That causes its own sort of stress and trauma," said Tweedy, who sometimes finds himself inundated with student concerns. "I think physician burnout among minorities in academic in medicine is very high." (The AAMC reported that Black or African-American doctors comprised 3.6 percent of medical school faculty in 2018, compared to 5 percent of working physicians or 8.4 percent of medical students.) Tweedy suggests that when medical schools are looking to diversify their faculty, they consider hiring more than one minority candidate at the same time so that they can share the workload when providing expertise and mentorship.

For healthcare workers in all capacities, adequate mentorship can make all the difference. After almost giving up on nursing after finding it abusive, unsafe, and unhealthy, Buffington transitioned into her "dream job" as an administrative nurse in Colorado and found a life coach who helped her overcome the "inner mean voice" that always told her she would fail. Now, she brings her sweet, engaging nature to counsel nurses around the country experiencing burnout through her consulting company, the Burnout Ward. She advises them to invest in self-preservation, such as adequate sleep and taking their scheduled breaks; as well as self-care, such as taking vacations, getting massages, and engaging in a hobby. As a recovering perfectionist, Buffington warns that it's also important to change one's mindset and avoid beating oneself up—as otherwise, self-care efforts will have little effect—while also standing up for oneself when necessary. "I think building resilience for nurses in particular is really about learning to advocate for themselves in the way they would advocate for a patient that is needing that additional support," she said.

Salt in the Wound

In addition to the self-preservation, self-care, and self-advocacy, healthcare workers benefit greatly from the support of peers, supervisors, and counselors. Such support can prove most necessary—and unfortunately, most lacking—following a bad patient outcome, particularly when an error is involved. Providers often feel guilty about losing a patient under the best of circumstances, so when a mistake occurs—whether it's caught quickly, has little effect, is damaging, or proves lethal—the experience can be traumatic. Due to the challenging nature of complex illnesses, glitches in the system, miscommunication, and other factors, medical error is, even for the best clinicians, not uncommon. A landmark report published by the Institute of Medicine in 2000 (now the National Academy of Medicine), "To Err is Human," suggested that medical error kills between 44,000 to 98,000 Americans every year, while a 2013 study from Johns Hopkins University (published in the *Journal of Patient Safety*) estimated that number to be between 210,000 to 440,000. The initial report also placed emphasis on the systemic nature of the healthcare industry as a main source of medical error, despite the US medical and legal systems' tradition of holding individuals responsible.

As a brand-new acute care nurse, Beth Hawkes was working in an orthopedic unit when a doctor ordered her to change the IV solution for an elderly patient. She did so—but, having heard wrong, she hung the new solution for the patient's roommate instead. Later that day, the nurse manager called Hawkes into her office. She had failed to check the patient's identity and, in hanging the IV, had committed two errors: both patients were receiving the wrong fluid. Hawkes was suspended for three days without pay. "It was shocking," she said. "I was worried that I'd harmed the patient. It was embarrassing because I was suspended. It was just kind of catastrophic, really."

Hawkes, who was used to being a top student, was confused and devastated. Fortunately, the patients hadn't suffered, but the mistake weighed on her for several months. It also made her much more careful. Hawkes, who's now a nursing professional development specialist for Adventist Health on the West Coast, and who spent a decade as a nurse manager, said she would have appreciated a more thorough investigation. "It was my fault, but I think it's really important to go, 'What really happened, what caused you to skip a step in a procedure or take a shortcut?'" she said. "I would have felt like somebody was striving to understand me."

When a clinician commits an obvious error, typically systemic factors contribute to the mistake. Albert Wu was participating in one of his very first codes as a physician-in-training when he was instructed to give morphine to a patient in heart failure. He administered five times more than required, and the patient went into respiratory arrest. Fortunately, the patient was rapidly intubated and resuscitated, but Wu felt shocked, distressed, ashamed, and guilty. "Fortunately, I got some support at that moment from an experienced nurse who happened to witness the whole thing," Wu said. The nurse reassured him and pointed out contributing factors in how the code was run. "It helped me to understand the incident in a slightly more objective way," Wu said.

Wu, who is now a professor of health policy and management at Johns Hopkins University, began researching medical error. Shortly after the Institute of Medicine report was published, he issued a short essay, "Medical Error: The Second Victim," which recognized the distress experienced by clinicians and called for sympathy and support rather than punitive measures. Wu has since established a program at Johns Hopkins called Resilience in Stressful Events (RISE), which provides peer support to clinicians following a bad outcome—whether an error was committed or not—by responding to a page within thirty minutes and then meeting to confidentially discuss the incident, usually that same day.

RISE began in 2011 with a team of eighteen peer supporters taking about one call a month and grew to thirty-five people by 2020. "I think the two most important things are actually showing up and listening," Wu said. Despite starting off slow, the fact that Johns Hopkins had the structure in place meant it was able to effectively respond to the pandemic—serving some 2,500 staff in the first three months, including food service workers and security guards—and also to other catastrophic incidents, such as when a patient's family member stabbed another family member to death. "Organizations need to appreciate that the places that they make people work are as high-risk in some ways as a construction site," Wu said. "And they need to plan proactively." The Maryland Patient Safety Center has since supported Johns Hopkins in establishing Caring for the Caregiver, which has trained some forty other health systems, mostly in the US, to develop programs similar to RISE.

While medical errors and other bad outcomes can be challenging for any practitioner, most physicians' greatest fear is the possibility of a malpractice claim—and for good reason. Stacia Dearmin, a pediatric emergency medicine physician in Ohio, was working at a community hospital when a young woman presented with an array of symptoms that fit a prior pattern and did not seem overly pressing. After observing her, running some tests, and discussing the young woman's case with her parents, Dearmin sent her home with the plan to follow up with her family doctor. The next day, Dearmin was shocked to learn that the young woman had been admitted to the ICU after suffering a respiratory arrest during which paramedics had been unable to establish an airway. Dearmin felt the way she did when a loved one died: "Time sort of stands still, and I feel like I'm outside my body, sort of a frozen sensation of disbelief," she said. "I just had this overwhelming feeling that I made the wrong choice."

The young woman died, and Dearmin turned to two mentors, including her medical director, both of whom assured her they wouldn't have done more; if anything, they told her, they would have done less. Still, Dearmin knew she'd likely be sued. Sure enough, she was—and for the three-and-a-half years from the patient's death until the lawsuit ended, the young woman weighed heavily on her mind, even as Dearmin continued to treat thousands of others. She experienced the sense of isolation so common to physicians engaged in litigation: the fear that she was a bad doctor, an imposter. The concern that hurting so much reflected negatively on her character. The inability to discuss the case with colleagues for fear of impinging on the legal process. After a crushing three-week trial, the jury reached a verdict in Dearmin's favor, and she was finally able to approach the patient's family and say how sorry she was—an action that, thanks to the parents' openness, provided as much relief as the verdict itself. Still, it was another three-and-a-half years before Dearmin began to feel like she'd recovered.

About a year after the patient's death, before the lawsuit had been filed, Dearmin came across Wu's article on the "second victim" and was strongly impacted by its suggestion that the physicians most susceptible to injury were also the most sensitive and reflective. "It was an enormous relief," Dearmin said. "I had a bad feeling about how long it was taking me to feel better, and I think I lacked the vocabulary for the experience." She watched a TED Talk about the epidemic of physician suicide, and while she wasn't suicidal, Dearmin found her own ordeal "so extraordinarily difficult" it became obvious to her that both adverse events and malpractice lawsuits, which can occur individually or simultaneously, were contributing factors. Afterward, Dearmin began doing some public speaking, beginning with her own division at the children's hospital where she now works—often, with her defense lawyer—and blogging about her experience. She now counsels physicians who are facing lawsuits and who often experience similar feelings of shame, guilt, anger, fear, and grief. Some begin to question their choice of career. "There's no reason why physicians should be so alone in this," Dearmin said.

While some 55 to 75 percent of physicians face malpractice lawsuits over the course of their careers, few are open about the experience. Louise Andrew, an internist and former emergency physician who spent thirteen years on faculty at Johns Hopkins University, was named in a malpractice suit as the supervising attending physician whose resident had sent home a patient who later died of unclear causes. "If a patient does badly, and you know about it or find out about it, you're already hurt. You already have a wound," Andrew said. To then face a malpractice suit, she said, is "like pouring in salt." The process can last for years, and often, just when a physician starts to relax or heal, a new piece of the litigation arises. "It's like a decubitus ulcer that can't possibly get better because pressure keeps getting put on," Andrew said. Nurses aren't immune to malpractice litigation, either: hundreds in the US are obligated to make malpractice payments every year.

In her book on medical error, *When We Do Harm: A Doctor Confronts Medical Error*, Danielle Ofri explored countries that have adopted alternative methods of addressing malpractice—such as Denmark, which provides monetary compensation to patients and family members for bad outcomes regardless of whether or not the doctor was at fault. Ofri, who disclosed her own challenges with medical error—including missing an anemia indicative of cancer, calling the wrong patient with good news about his blood sugar, and entering the wrong patient language when adapting to changes in the electronic medical record—recognized that while it could be immensely traumatic for patients and their families, doctors were also affected, even when not facing allegations of malpractice. "For doctors and nurses, it's devastating to have missed a serious diagnosis, and agonizing to contemplate the additional stress you've caused your patient, above and beyond the illness itself," she wrote. Meanwhile, physicians who face malpractice claims despite performing to the highest standards are significantly distressed by long, drawn-out court proceedings that question their integrity and competence.

Following her lawsuit, Andrew obtained a law degree, which she uses to counsel physicians on the legal, emotional, and practical aspects of their cases, including those to whom they can safely speak about the experience and how to maintain healthy sleep and exercise patterns while preparing for trial. Many physicians, she said, subsequently end up putting up walls because they begin to see all patients as potential plaintiffs and become wary of showing any signs of imperfection. Studies have shown that as many as three-quarters of specialists view their patients as potential litigants, while those who've already been sued are more likely to practice medicine defensively, as well as to face further litigation. "It's actually a grief-producing situation, and for some doctors, it's career-ending," said Andrew, whose long-standing interest in physician well-being has been profoundly influenced by her own family's history with depression and suicide. "With all physicians, you can work to heal the trauma; but most of us, sadly, are never the same again after a malpractice claim."

"Took Me Over the Edge"

For doctors facing the fallout of malpractice claims, cumulative trauma, or other significant stressors, an inability to adaptively respond to the issue can permanently end their careers. Legal action was a significant factor in John Danyi's attempted suicide, followed by the loss of his thirty-year career as a highly-regarded anesthesiologist—despite the fact that he did nothing wrong. After working as chief of anesthesia in both California and Virginia, Danyi and his business partner, also an anesthesiologist, contracted with a surgery center in Virginia. Then, his partner lost a patient on the operating table during a carpal tunnel surgery. Following a second incident involving his partner, the surgery center declined to work with her further, and in the process of dissolving the joint corporation she held with Danyi, she sued Danyi for failing to protect her business interests. "That legal hassle was enormous," said Danyi, who ended up paying hundreds of thousands of dollars to settle the case, while also taking on the role of medical director at the surgery center and creating policies to ensure the situation wouldn't occur again. Danyi, who was going through a difficult divorce at the same time, became increasingly depressed. Then, he brought on a new partner who immediately took ill, and when Danyi suggested that she cover for him on her return so that he could take some time off, she told him he should "just retire already." Danyi began to question whether his existence was even useful. "The last thing I had was my identity as a physician, as an anesthesiologist," he said. "That was the thing that took me over the edge."

Late one night in July 2017, Danyi wrote emails to several family members and friends to "assuage any guilt that they might feel that they'd missed something" and injected a fatal dose of Fentanyl. But one person he'd written in Australia, who was awake due to the time difference, alerted the authorities. Danyi was surprised to find himself regaining consciousness in the ICU, where his first thought was, "Why did they put IVs in my elbow?"—a complaint typical of anesthesiologists. The second was: "I wonder why I survived." Deciding that there must be a purpose for his continued existence, Danyi determined to pull himself out of his depression and was compliant with his therapy, including a "fairly humiliating" week-plus at a psychiatric inpatient facility followed by a referral to the Virginia Health Practitioners Monitoring Program (HPMP).

Danyi said that the surgery center not only refused to take him back after his suicide attempt but also requested that he resign his staff privileges while under investigation by the Virginia Board of Medicine—severely impairing his employability. "What I've learned is that once you've attempted suicide, you're viewed as damaged goods," Danyi said. The medical board handed him over to the state monitoring program, which required him to sign a five-year contract and submit to measures such as regular therapy, drug screening, and attending Alcoholics Anonymous meetings—even though he had no history of substance abuse. Their requirements also made it difficult for Danyi to take outdoor excursions to go camping or whitewater rafting, which Danyi considered ludicrous and antitherapeutic. In October 2018, Danyi decided to move to Oregon, where he found the state physician health program much more reasonable and supportive. (The Federation of State Physician Health Programs did not respond to emails seeking comment on the differences between state programs.) Danyi, who no longer suffers from depression, still hasn't been able to obtain insurance to practice anesthesia due to his extended absence from the field but has rediscovered a sense of purpose by opening a clinic that provides ketamine therapy to people with depression, PTSD, and suicidal ideation—serving numerous healthcare workers during the COVID-19 pandemic.

Burnout and trauma weigh heavily on doctors and other health-care workers and, when coupled with depression, personal tragedies, litigation, or other stressors, can easily become life-threatening. A 2018 analysis of peer-reviewed literature over the previous decade found that physicians commit suicide at a rate of 28 to 40 per 100,000, more than double the 12.3 per 100,000 in the general population. Pamela Wible, an internal medicine doctor in Oregon, began documenting physician suicides on her blog after attending the third memorial service for a doctor in her small town in 2012 and counted more than 860 in the US after six years—a startling number that continues to rise. "I wanted to know why," wrote Wible, who found that anesthesiologists are more than twice as likely to die by suicide than physicians in any other specialty. Surgeons had the second highest numbers, followed by emergency medicine physicians, obstetricians/gynecologists, and psychiatrists.

Danyi said that physicians in general struggle with the amount of pain and suffering they encounter, while anesthesiologists are repeatedly exposed to trauma in the operating room. He recalled one of his first patients in California, a man who was moving a refrigerator downstairs with his friend when it fell on him. The patient was awake and talking when Danyi sedated him, but after surgeons opened up his abdomen, they found that his vena cava was irreparably torn and there was nothing they could do. "If you've not spent a lifetime dealing with trauma vicariously, it's hard to imagine what that's like," he said. "Let me tell you this: it's a stress."

Emergency medical technicians and other first responders also encounter inordinate amounts of trauma and suffer disproportionately high rates of suicide: one study in Arizona, published in *Prehospital Emergency Care*, found that 5.6 percent of EMT deaths were categorized as suicide from 2009–2015, compared to 2.2 percent in the general population. First responders receive much less recognition—and not nearly as much compensation—as doctors and nurses, yet witness the same level of trauma, death, and suffering. Meanwhile, they're afforded less opportunity to process such occurrences. Due to the short period of time they spend with patients, their grief remains highly disenfranchised, and they're rarely involved in debriefings, huddles, or similar methods of decompression employed in hospital settings. And they're fearful of seeking help: Alexandra Jabr, the firefighter and paramedic educator in California, said that in addition to the stigma, first responders in her state are rarely willing to reach out when having suicidal thoughts because those who do could be placed on a "5150"—the California legal code for temporary, involuntary psychiatric commitment.

Jabr regularly takes phone calls from first responders who are suffering from insomnia, or who are depressed, drunk, or suicidal, such as the friend who'd responded to a "really bad, just disgusting call" involving the death of a child, and told her that he couldn't sleep for the first time in twelve years, that every single call in which a patient had died had been resurfacing to plague him. "That's the thing about trauma in this field, and PTSD, is that it's cumulative," Jabr said. "You stay quiet about it, and then it gets pushed down, it never gets processed, and it never gets resolved. And then guess what—it's years later and it's coming to visit you." Jabr noted that while individual responses can depend as much on someone's life situation and state of mind as on the nature of the call or past experience, it's always hard to predict who will be impacted and why. Just after submitting the application for her master's degree, Jabr heard that a former paramedic colleague, someone she'd worked with closely for two years in Orange County, had committed suicide—an outcome she'd never anticipated. "There's so much more involved than just a bad call," she said.

Jabr would like to see more first responders taking advantage of counseling services such as cognitive behavioral therapy, as well as improving sleep hygiene, food choices, and other behavioral habits. While concerned by the high rate of suicides, she's equally disturbed by the prevalence of substance abuse and other negative coping mechanisms—particularly alcohol, which was once her drug of choice. "How about the ones that are killing themselves slowly?" she said. "How about the ones that don't care whether or not they get a DUI and hit somebody? They're the people that are literally just not thriving because of all of these events happening in their lives."

Studies are inconclusive as to whether physicians are more likely to abuse substances than the general population, but the availability of prescription medication does create a unique temptation for those under stress. Lou Ortenzio, a former family physician, was so committed to his patients in the small town of Clarksburg, West Virginia, that he would sometimes extend his hours until 11:30 p.m. at night to provide each of them with personalized care. "I did not have a very good sense of limits or boundaries," said Ortenzio, who began overprescribing opioids to his patients when they asked. Soon, he started taking them himself—Tylenol-with-codeine and Darvocet at first; then, Hydrocodone. "I overbooked myself and overscheduled myself and overworked myself," he said. "When the stress of it all mounted up, I could abuse opiates. And they were like magic." Initially, Ortenzio pocketed samples handed out by pharmaceutical reps, but he then began asking patients to fill prescriptions for him and wrote fraudulent prescriptions in his children's names. Toward the end, he was popping thirty to forty pills a day—a toxic dose of Tylenol. "I just didn't see any way that I could quit," Ortenzio said. "Patients depended on me. I thought my family depended on me. I had an office staff that I had to support." Eventually, it was Ortenizo's office staff that stepped in to stage an intervention; at the same time, a nurse introduced him to Jesus. Somehow, with the support and prayers of everyone involved, Ortenzio managed to get clean in a few days, without treatment. Later, after federal agents raided his office and Ortenzio lost his license, his marriage, and his reputation, he was grateful for the widespread community support that kept him out of jail; instead, he received a supervised release, a fine, and community service. He worked as a golf course greenskeeper, a pizza delivery person, and an office supply salesman, eventually marrying the nurse who introduced him to his faith and becoming the executive director of the Clarksburg Mission, where he now serves the homeless and those suffering from mental health and substance abuse issues. Ortenzio, who receives a phone call roughly once month from doctors or nurses struggling with substance issues, whom he refers to the state physician health program, advises those considering opioids or other substances to ask for help. "Have as many supporting friends as you can confide in," he said. "Cultivate relationships early on with people outside the medical field. Develop a hobby, although it seems difficult." Ortenzio, who would have appreciated more discussion of boundaries and limits in medical training, believes he would have been better off if he hadn't seen himself as the ultimate authority. Now, he has God. "I was kind of a lone ranger, and you can't be a lone ranger," he said.

While burnout in all specialties can lead to substance abuse, depression, or even suicide, those exposed to trauma are burdened with that additional stress, as well as the potential to blame themselves for bad outcomes. Michael Weinstein, a trauma surgeon in Philadelphia who's struggled with depression since he was a teenager, took an indefinite leave from surgery in October 2018 after suffering a "really tough loss" in the operating room. He'd tried to help his partner, who was experiencing difficulty during an elective surgery, and the patient died. "It was really challenging for me, perhaps more than others, and no one really wanted to talk about it other than kind of the medical facts," he said.

Because this wasn't the first time that Weinstein had succumbed to depression on the job, he knew to address it early. In 2016, after months of wanting to get help but fearing the stigma and embarrassment associated with mental health issues, Weinstein submitted himself to elective inpatient electroconvulsive therapy. He became suicidal and was institutionalized. After some time—thanks to the support of his wife and children, cognitive behavioral therapy, effective medication, and mindfulness practices—Weinstein recovered and returned to practice. But following his most recent experience with a patient's death, and the lack of any support for its emotional impact, Weinstein felt he "just couldn't return to that world."

Since leaving surgery, Weinstein has been providing primary care for Project HOME, an organization that serves the poor and homeless in Philadelphia, and developing a support program for physicians and other clinicians. But in Spring 2020, as the COVID-19 pandemic froze much of that activity and his mental health worsened, his efforts stalled. "I'm hoping that my recovery trajectory is still on its way up," said Weinstein, who engages in meditation and yoga and tries to focus on where he finds meaning and purpose—such as with his family, and by helping others. "It's just day by day, hour by hour." Weinstein said that while working in trauma surgery sometimes provided a distraction from his depression, it could also be exhausting, as he was often on call. "I think it was just the accumulation of not ever feeling like I was performing as well as I should, working, not ever saying no, and taking on different leadership, administrative tasks," he said. "And when I see people suffering, it affects me. There's a spectrum of that sensitivity and empathy that could be better honored and supported."

Part II

Rediscovering
Medicine's Humanity

5

Creating Space for Grief and Trauma

There is some strange intimacy between grief and aliveness,
some sacred exchange between what seems unbearable and
what is most exquisitely alive.

—FRANCIS WELLER

Children mangled by car accidents, young mothers succumbing to cancer, unexpected deaths in the operating room: the list of traumas experienced by medical professionals is long and varied. Many healthcare workers find themselves deeply affected by their patients' tragic circumstances and shoulder an increasingly heavy burden of unresolved grief. But these days, they are beginning to embrace innovative ways of coping. Perhaps surprisingly, many of these efforts involve finding greater connection with patients who are dying, as well as seeking support from therapists, chaplains, and the larger faith community. By recognizing and honoring the humanity of those they serve, healthcare professionals find that they are able to mitigate their own feelings of distress about the suffering and death they're forced to witness daily.

While popular television programs including *ER* and *Grey's Anatomy* portray doctors and nurses as heroic figures rushing in to save the majority of their patients' lives, the reality is much bleaker. More than 650,000 people die of heart disease in the US every year, while nearly 600,000 die of cancer, according to the Centers for Disease Control and Prevention (CDC). Meanwhile, tens of thousands die from stroke, respiratory diseases, Alzheimer's disease, diabetes, and other conditions. For many, death comes after long and painful battles with illness, which can make extraordinary measures at the end of life even more heartbreaking.

When CPR is applied under such circumstances, it rarely succeeds: of the 290,000-plus adults who suffer from cardiac arrest in US hospitals each year, less than 20 percent are fortunate enough to be discharged—meaning only around 58,000 survive. Efforts to resuscitate a patient suffering cardiac or respiratory arrest—known as "code blues"—are made even more traumatic by the violent nature of their performance and prove particularly challenging when involving older, or seriously ill, patients. "If CPR is done right, it breaks your ribs and your sternum," said Marilyn Reiss-Carradero, a rapid response nurse at an urban California hospital who participates in as many as a dozen code blues a year. "Especially when you're working on somebody that is elderly, truly we feel like we are torturing or contributing to a very violent death." During the procedure, doctors and nurses work to obtain IV access through a patient's legs and arms, while others insert a breathing tube down the patient's throat or administer shocks from a defibrillator to restart the heart—causing their body to literally jump. "The first time you see that, that's an image you just don't forget," Reiss-Carradero said.

Jessica Zitter, a pulmonary critical care and palliative care–trained physician at Oakland's Highland Hospital and author of *Extreme Measures: Finding a Better Path to the End of Life*, regularly experiences the trauma of code blues and acknowledges that it's not always easy to manage the emotions involved—particularly for terminally ill patients who, if they survive, may only suffer more. "To witness, and frankly even to know that you're contributing to, suffering in a person, you don't feel the compassion because you avoid it," Zitter said. "You move away from it—it's too painful to witness, particularly if you feel you've played a role in it. And so you withdraw further, and that's extremely distressing and numbing. Numbing is a way of managing it and surviving it."

When Samuel Slavin was a student at Harvard Medical School, he interviewed a range of hospital staff for a Transom radio piece called "Anatomy of a Code Blue" and found that all were deeply affected by the trauma of code blues, no matter what their role. "It's interesting thinking back to making 'Anatomy of a Code Blue' as a medical student, and then being involved in many more of those situations as a doctor," said Slavin in his final year of residency at Massachusetts General Hospital. "It's something that is devastating and has a powerful impact on us, and is also something that is relatively routine and part of a day's work."

Slavin has since participated in somewhere between twenty to thirty code blues. As a senior resident, he's responsible for running the code, which he said puts additional pressure on a doctor's ego that can make processing such situations even more challenging. "Even though we know that most of the time the doctor is not someone swooping in to make a brilliant save, and we also know very much that it is a team effort, especially when things go right," he said, "there's a big part of me that wants to be a brilliant leader." Slavin said it's hard not to place expectations on himself to create a calm and controlled situation, one that best serves the patient. "When things don't turn out well, you wonder why," he said. "I'll find myself beating myself up for days before I take a step back and tease apart what are those things that I actually could have done better, and what are the things that were actually outside of my control."

The entire healthcare team, from surgeons to janitorial staff, is affected by the trauma of code blues. In the Transom radio piece, Marie, a long-term member of the housekeeping staff told Slavin: "After a code I could compare it to, if you've seen a tornado, afterward everything is strewn and everything is smashed." She added, "You find some rooms that don't have much on the floor—it makes me think, maybe that person survived? What am I thinking? I'm thinking, God—let this person live."

"A Sacred Moment"

Fortunately, some healthcare workers have been stepping up to restore meaning and ritual to the death process. Roughly a decade ago, Jonathan Bartels was working as a trauma nurse in the University of Virginia Health System when he was inspired by a chaplain who asked everyone to stop after a patient's death and said a prayer. While Bartels didn't relate to the religious nature of her prayer, he was struck by the power of the concept, and translated it into "the Medical Pause," which uses secular language to call for a moment of silence. "You can have someone who's Christian next to someone who's Hindu next to someone who's Buddhist, and someone who's atheist or agnostic, all honoring that patient but doing it in silence," he said. "But all with the same mission—which is really to take a moment to recognize this last rite of passage. To reinstate ritual, or a ritual, back into a system that has driven ritual out through its scientific pursuits."

Bartels said that he witnessed an immediate difference when experiencing the trauma of code blues and other patient deaths. "I didn't just separate, I was able to close the gap from one act to another, and I was able to put [the trauma] down," he said. "And then my peers were able to put it down. But it's not—and I say this often—it's not a panacea, it's not a cure-all. This is the first step in many, many steps of what is really being called for to take care of ourselves."

Since then, Bartels said that hospital professionals from New Mexico, Cleveland, Washington state—even as far away as South Africa—have reached out for advice in implementing similar practices. Reiss-Carradero was motivated to introduce a "Moment of Silence" at her hospital, during which staff recognize the patient by name, after reading about it in a journal article. "Just acknowledging that this is a sacred moment for that patient," she said. "Because that's what's lost in a code blue death—there is nothing spiritual, there's nothing comforting, there's nothing calm and quiet." Reiss-Carradero also began to take additional, personal steps, like covering the patient. "Now, I make sure that I touch them in some way," she said. "Whether that's holding their hand—it depends where I am in the room, if it's crowded—or I touch their forehead."

As Bartels found, ritual doesn't need to be elaborate to be effective. "The biggest difference was the way people left that room," Bartels said. While clinicians will typically toss their gloves on the floor, along with the equipment and blood, and walk out, the Pause allowed them to reconnect and leave with a sense of reverence. "This really changed things because we could stop to honor that person, and not walk away disappointed," he said.

Other hospitals have begun similar efforts to recognize organ donors, known as *honor walks*, in which doctors, nurses and other hospital staff line the hallway as a recently deceased patient is wheeled into the operating room. LifeCenter Organ Donor Network in Cincinnati began implementing the practice at their thirty-five Cincinnati-area hospitals in December of 2017 after a survey indicated that staff wanted to be more involved. Anywhere from four to one hundred friends and family members can show up for the event, which occurs at various times of day or night—whenever the patient is scheduled into the operating room. And when LifeCenter posted a photograph taken by family members of one donor to Facebook, it went viral—inspiring still others, including Jennifer DeMaroney, organ donation coordinator at the University of Vermont Medical Center.

"It's so striking," said DeMaroney, who has since consulted with an estimated one hundred hospitals on the practice. "I knew that at our hospital, this would be something that they would get really excited about." DeMaroney was right. Her hospital instituted honor walks shortly after and encouraged families to personalize the experience. Many tape photographs of their loved one to the bed—often picturing them doing activities they enjoyed, such as hunting or fishing. One family held a Native American drumming ceremony, while another brought in their entire church gospel choir to sing throughout the process. For one elementary-aged girl, most of her class showed up to participate. "It's bringing awareness, but it is also supporting the staff that are taking care of the donor and their family, because these cases are hard on everyone," DeMaroney said. "People will tell you where they were when they saw their first honor walk, how it affected them."

Such moments are powerful. Zitter vividly recalls the first time she witnessed an ER resident implement a moment of silence following a patient's death. It was only a few years ago—something the resident had been taught in her training. "I was blown away," Zitter said. "I was so touched, and moved, and I thought, why haven't we done this before? This is exactly what we need to do when a person's life passes through your hands." Since then, Zitter has continued the practice. "This is very big stuff, and it should be meaningful," she said. "The second we stop seeing it as meaningful and human and poignant and sad and connecting, that's when we start to lose our humanity."

Bridging the Gap

For many healthcare workers, chaplains and other members of the faith community provide essential support—not only to bring in the sacred, but also to connect with patients, to process emotions, and to navigate challenging circumstances. Zitter said that collaborating with other staff on her palliative care team, including a nurse, social worker, and chaplain, has helped her forge stronger bonds with patients. "We learn how to connect with people in ways that we didn't learn in typical medical school classes," she said. "Working with chaplains and social workers who already learn this in a different way in their education, we in the palliative care movement tend to be better and less agenda-driven at sort of forging an interaction and connection with somebody than is typical."

Zitter has also been partnering with faith leaders in Oakland to bridge the gap in understanding between healthcare providers and underserved communities—such as Rev. Cynthia Carter Perrilliat, executive director of the Alameda County Care Alliance (ACCA). Through its Advanced Illness Care Program (AICP), the organization links people with advanced illness and their caregivers to trusted resources, assisting the predominantly African-American community to navigate—and establish effective communication with—the healthcare system. "They speak different languages," said Perrilliat, who is also minister of civic partnerships at Allen Temple Baptist Church. "The onus is frankly on the medical community to prepare themselves and to have the cultural sensitivity and humility to get to understand the people that they're caring for." The program—which brings physicians together with pastors for informal dinners, and sometimes invites a facilitator to lead discussions—has proved popular in both cohorts. "Faith leaders are keepers not only of the faith, but keepers of traditions within communities," said Perrilliat, who compared their role to that of family physicians in the past, when they would make house calls and walk with their patients from the cradle to the grave. "The community, and the faith-based community in particular, is really uniquely positioned to bridge the gap with health systems."

Support from pastoral care is also what gets some physicians, nurses, and other healthcare staff through their most difficult moments. Tyler Hughes, who spent more than two decades as the general surgeon for a rural community in McPherson, Kansas, was often impacted by the fact that he knew his patients personally and found some situations harder to handle than others—such as the patient who died unexpectedly during a gallbladder operation. "I was able to compartmentalize when things went wrong," said Hughes, who'd developed the skill set to deal with the occasional bad outcomes during his twelve years of prior practice in Dallas and had learned coping mechanisms after losing his own child in infancy. "But that didn't mean that I didn't think about it, occasionally brood about it, and then ask for help from my associate who's a surgeon." Hughes added that he always knew that if things became especially difficult, he could reach out to his pastor. "I was fortunate to have a good relationship with a pastor who was a professionally trained counselor, so we could talk," he said.

More formally, chaplains are present in hospitals, hospices, and long-term care settings to provide spiritual care to patients and families, as well as to assist in conversations around goals at the end of life. Yet while healthcare organizations such as hospitals and nursing homes have been required since the 1960s to provide spiritual or religious support to patients, in recent years the role of chaplains has expanded to extend social, spiritual, and emotional support to nurses, doctors, and other medical professionals. In many settings—particularly in hospice and palliative care, or at critical decision-making moments in the ICU—chaplains are considered vital members of the interdisciplinary healthcare team. They will often participate in debriefings, check in with staff, and organize memorials to commemorate patient deaths.

For many clinicians, connecting with hospital chaplains at pivotal moments can help to shift their perspective. Khurram Ahmed, a chaplain at Stony Brook University Hospital on Long Island, New York, began his training in 2014 after he became disillusioned by watching the race riots in Ferguson, Missouri, on television. He was unsettled by how common it was for Black men to be targeted by police; how distanced our society had become from its humanity. He was considering joining the police force when his wife, an ICU physician, suggested he speak with the chaplain at her hospital—and the encounter proved life-changing. "He had the ability to hold the space where everybody can feel supported, feel dignified, feel heard, feel respected," Ahmed said. "So if those are tools that I hope to introduce to these contexts that we're seeing, then this is probably as good a place as any to start." Ahmed now facilitates the Muslim jama'ah prayer at Stony Brook while also helping patients from diverse religious and cultural backgrounds to identify and communicate goals of care, and offering "support for whatever the patient, or the family member, or the staff member, is going through."

One powerful instance of his ability to do so occurred in the midst of the COVID-19 crisis, when the hospital was housing some four hundred confirmed or suspected cases. Ahmed was in the hospital lobby, waiting for the elevator, when a physician shared that she was thinking about quitting. "I don't think I can do this," she told him. They discussed her thoughts of returning to Florida, and what was stopping her, including concerns about traveling so far with her elderly dog. Ahmed asked her how she felt about her choice to prioritize the dog, and she began to view the situation in a different light. "It's the right decision," she told him. "I'm happy with that." While the conversation didn't touch on religion, or the challenges of her work, or the virus, it allowed the doctor to establish a more positive framework that embraced her continued commitment.

Sensei Koshin Paley Ellison, a Zen teacher and chaplaincy educator, has witnessed many such turning points. Ellison became a chaplain when, after caring for his grandmother in his early twenties, she asked him to use his skills to help others at the end of life. "She said, 'There's just something to the Zen thing,'" Ellison recalled. So along with his partner, Robert Chodo Campbell, Ellison enrolled in a chaplaincy training program, and in 2007, the duo co-founded the New York Zen Center for Contemplative Care.

Ellison takes a rather Zen approach to his role, which he describes as being "to dwell and to rest in what I don't know, which is most things, and to be deeply curious." In approaching patients, or when supporting hospital staff, Ellison finds it most important to be deeply present and grounded in his body through their basic meditation posture—an upright stature, with shoulders back, and a softness in the belly two inches below the navel. "My great wish in terms of training chaplains is to get them to feel really in their bodies, really grounded in their softness, so that they can widen out and be connected to what matters most," he said.

In addition to training programs, the center has recently been working with hospitals, hospices, and nursing homes to provide contemplative-based resilience training, using a unique curriculum that focuses on meaning, agency, and connection. Participants, who can range from doctors to janitorial staff, typically start with a contemplation and meditation before engaging in group discussions. During an eight-week resiliency training for attending physicians, Ellison said that one OB-GYN, who'd been practicing for thirty years and was so burned out she said she'd "crawled" into the training, realized that she hadn't looked a patient in the eye since she started her residency. The reason was that during that residency, she'd had to tell a pregnant mother that her seven-month-old unborn baby had died. "She had no training for that conversation, and so she just stopped looking at patients," Ellison said, adding that by working together, the physician was able to renew her sense of connection. "She started to feel, both for herself and for patients, completely transformed," he said.

Joseph Perez, vice president of mission and ministry at Valley Baptist Health, who has spent many years as a chaplain in hospice, outpatient, and inpatient settings, said he works to support hospital staff as much as possible during such moments of difficulty. One way he does that is to offer to include them when praying for a patient—whether that is going into surgery or following a patient's death. "I allude to the idea of a journey," said Perez, who oversees chaplaincy services at two hospitals in Harlingen and Brownsville, Texas, including around eighteen staff and forty volunteers. "We're all walking this path together. And I think it's something that breeds a sense of wholeness and health. It fights the idea of isolation and being alone, of course, and it also recognizes that not one person can do everything. That it takes a community of people to do this well." Perez said he'll often follow up with doctors and nurses following a code blue or other challenging event—to check on them, affirm their effort, and acknowledge the hardship they've gone through.

Respiratory therapist Lufta Bana said the chaplain at her hospital, a Level 1 Trauma Center in Columbus, Ohio, has helped her navigate many such emotional traumas. When Bana arrives to intubate patients, family members often have difficult questions about how long their loved one will live. And when she extubates those who haven't recovered, Bana facilitates their death. "The last thing they see would be me pulling that tube and turning the machine off," said Bana, who sometimes sees multiple deaths per shift. "It's hard." Bana particularly struggles with performing this task in the neonatal ICU. "There's no rationality," she said of infant deaths. "That's when I go home crying."

Bana appreciates the single chaplain available on the twelve-hour night shifts she works three days a week. Though he's often busy, he checks in with her in passing, engages her in more meaningful conversation when things are slow, and follows up after a difficult code. "You can just deal with it, say what you're feeling, and just move on," Bana said, "instead of having to process all of that at the end of a long shift." While the chaplain is a Christian and Bana is a Muslim, that hasn't prevented her from benefiting from his services. "He really talks to us equally," said

Bana, who would nevertheless appreciate the opportunity to have chaplains from other religions on duty, even if only once a month.

Perez, who was formerly the president of the Association of Professional Chaplains (APC), said he's also found it imperative to acknowledge difficult emotions and find ways to embrace and process the sadness. "I've learned so much from the dying," he said. "To learn how to carry sadness is really important—grief is a part of that, and mourning is part of that. Sadness deepens our heart. It helps us to go to deep places in our heart, and when we run away from sadness, we actually stop ourselves from growing. We have to learn that sadness is actually the flip side of happiness or joy. And if we don't go deep with the sadness, we can't go deep with the happiness, either." In this spirit, Perez makes himself available to staff, patients, and families as necessary.

For Rabbi Bryan Kinzbrunner, director of religious and spiritual services at The Oscar and Ella Wilf Campus for Senior Living, a Jewish residential community in Somerset, New Jersey, that includes assisted living, independent living, and hospice, supporting staff expressions of grief and hardship also means determining when they're ready—and sometimes, that's well after the traumatic experience has passed. When a staff support session in the midst of the COVID-19 pandemic received a lukewarm response, Kinzbrunner realized they'd made the effort too early on. "The time to grieve is not in the middle of a battle," Kinzbrunner said. "I think that what's going to happen is ultimately there will be a lot of work to be done down the road when this is over."

As one of the community's two hospice chaplains, Kinzbrunner's multifaceted role involves buttressing patients, family members, and staff who are navigating challenging questions around quality of life, goals of care, and the death process. He plays a key role in family meetings, serving as a patient advocate while also bringing a sense of calmness to the room. "A good chaplain will know how to balance those things," said Kinzbrunner, who is president of the Neshama: Association of Jewish Chaplains (NAJC), and has some fifteen years of experience. "When you have a meeting like that and a chaplain is present, it often changes the dynamic." Kinzbrunner said he'll assist family engaging with existential questions—such as why their loved one has to suffer, or why the dying process has to take so long—while also supporting the staff. "One of the chaplain's roles is to listen to the team as they're going through their struggles with being around people who are dying all the time," he said. "It takes its toll on everybody, no matter how veteran one is."

"In the Middle of a Crisis"

Meanwhile, individuals and organizations have begun advocating for better access to mental healthcare for medical professionals, who continue to face significant hurdles to care despite high suicide rates, substance abuse, and other maladaptive tendencies. Healthcare workers are hardly alone: neuropsychiatric disorders have been cited as the leading underlying reason for disability within the United States. Worldwide, the World Health Organization (WHO) has identified such disorders to be responsible for 30.8 percent of years lived with disability. Yet for healthcare practitioners juggling personal issues along with immense responsibility, long hours, patient deaths, and mounds of paperwork, mental health services can be shockingly hard to access. Depending on their state and institution, doctors, nurses, and other healthcare workers confront a variety of hurdles that can put their reputations, their careers, and even their lives at risk.

Many state medical licensing boards require doctors and nurses to disclose treatment for mental illness—work-related or otherwise—with some states asking significantly more invasive questions than others. Those who answer in the affirmative can be submitted to a detailed analysis of their confidential health records in order to be deemed fit for practice and may even be penalized. A 2016 Mayo Clinic study of state medical initial licensure and renewal applications found that only one-third of US states in each category are considered "consistent," meaning that they only asked about current impairment from a mental health condition or didn't ask about mental health conditions at all. In addition, nearly 40 percent of physicians reported reluctance to seek mental health treatment for fear of licensure repercussions, with fewer reporting reluctance in states with a consistent ranking.

According to Pamela Wible, author of *Physician Suicide Letters—Answered* who co-authored a 2019 analysis of states' mental health questions and their impact, "state boards, even health plan and malpractice insurance companies, interrogate doctors about their mental health, read their confidential medical records, and then deny health plan participation, medical liability coverage, hospital privileges, and state licensure." Meanwhile, a 2019 study of nursing licensure questions published in the *Journal of Psychosocial Nursing and Mental Health Services* found that out of a total of thirty state boards who actually asked mental health questions, only eight of them contained questions regarded as legitimately legal under the Americans with Disabilities Act. While some states—including California and Florida—have recently taken action to review or address these issues, many of these standards remain in place. And as a result, doctors and nurses suffering from depression, anxiety, PTSD, or suicidal thoughts are much less likely than the average person to seek support for fear of endangering their careers.

In addition, some doctors seeking mental health services find themselves referred to controversial physician health programs (PHPs)—such as the one anesthesiologist John Danyi encountered after attempting suicide—which can require them to pay for lengthy and expensive rehabilitation treatments, undergo rigorous psychological evaluations, and submit to witnessed urine testing, whether or not they have substance abuse issues. One former medical doctor, Melissa Freeman, published an article in the journal *Qualitative Research in Medicine and Healthcare* in 2019 detailing how obtaining antidepressants and anxiety medication from a psychiatrist and suboptimal patient satisfaction scores caused her to be referred to the Washington state PHP (WPHP), and eventually, to quit her job and lose her license. A lawyer for WPHP disagreed with her narrative, saying in an emailed statement that "while WPHP would never violate Freeman's confidentiality in defending itself against such misrepresentations, WPHP believes that it is important, for the sake of those who need PHP services, that it goes on record to state clearly that the narrative in this article is false." Meanwhile, Linda Bresnahan, executive director of the Federation of State Physician Health Programs (FSPHP), pointed to positive participant stories, posted anonymously on FSPHP's website, as well as research, much of which was PHP-affiliated, that found the programs had high recovery rates for doctors with both mental health and substance abuse issues. (She did not respond to specific questions seeking comment.) "To avoid punishment by PHPs and boards (that may restrict licensure and publish doctors' mental health diagnoses online) physicians drive hundreds of miles out of town, use fake names, and pay cash for off-the-grid care," Wible wrote in the 2019 paper.

Elisabeth Poorman, an internal medicine physician who serves as chair of the wellness committee for the King County Medical Society in Washington state, said she's "counseled many people in places that actively punish you for seeking therapy or asking for help." Poorman has become a voice and resource for physicians seeking mental health services since speaking up about the major depressive episode she experienced during her residency on the East Coast. "It was difficult to find help that felt safe, that felt like my privacy would be protected," said Poorman, who found that her institution, while supportive, directed her to treatment within the building that she didn't feel comfortable attending. "At the same time I was being told that what I was experiencing was normal, everybody felt this way, when it seemed quite clear to me that I was depressed." Poorman wasn't able to secure effective help for nearly a year, and when another intern jumped off the building where she was staying—one of three who committed suicide that summer—she felt she had to speak up. "Once I started talking publicly about it, people started coming to me because they're so desperate for anybody that feels safe," Poorman said.

Now several years later, Poorman counsels physicians nationwide on where and how to safely access mental health services. "Institutions need to do a lot more work to destigmatize mental illness," Poorman said. "And then secondly, to acknowledge that people have a legitimate reason to be paranoid." Poorman advocates creating a "rigorously private access to care," as well as "reminding everybody how common this is, and that our aversion to seeking help for a medical illness is a kind of insanity."

Stephanie Zerwas, a psychologist and associate professor of psychiatry at the University of North Carolina at Chapel Hill, is a proponent of the university's "Taking Care of Our Own" program that assesses healthcare workers' wellness over time and provides feedback. As the COVID-19 pandemic hit, in mid-March of 2020, Zerwas worked with a friend to expand their services by reaching out to local therapists; within four days, some ninety had volunteered to provide virtual pro bono care through what they named Project Parachute. Soon, requests were pouring in from around the country asking how to implement similar telehealth programs, and Zerwas began matching people on her own. "I was quickly becoming overwhelmed," she said. "I started to realize that I was going to be the bottleneck."

Fortunately, a colleague connected Zerwas to Eleos Health, a digital mental health intelligence company that agreed to collaborate, and they quickly built a website. Some five months later, Project Parachute had matched more than three hundred physicians, residents, administrators, and other healthcare professionals to therapists within their state—and was considering expanding services to healthcare workers' family members. "Healthcare professionals tend to be really stoic, and also really selfless," Zerwas said. "They often will bottle up some really difficult stories because they're just worried that their loved ones or their friends won't want to hear it and can't tolerate it." While more than six hundred therapists joined the program, Zerwas said there had been fewer clinicians, likely due to stigma and fear of professional repercussions. (More than six months into the pandemic, one poll by the American College of Emergency Physicians [ACEP] found that 45 percent of emergency doctors didn't feel comfortable seeking mental health treatment for these reasons despite increased levels of stress and burnout.) "It definitely gives people pause," Zerwas said.

Jessica Gold, an assistant professor of psychiatry at Washington University School of Medicine in St. Louis, Missouri—who provides mental health services mostly to medical students but also sees residents and physicians as well as patients—agrees that a more open and honest discussion is required. Gold, who first became interested in doctor and student wellness after watching people drop out of her pre-med program in college, said there needs to be a cultural change in how mental health services are accessed, discussed, and provided in educational, training, and workplace settings. "It needs to be something that's inherently built in throughout all of these experiences," said Gold, pointing out that residents who see a physician dismiss a patient's depression might feel that their own would be discounted if revealed. Access to services should also be more available, better promoted, and covered, Gold said—without making healthcare workers feel that they're leaving other staff in the lurch if they attend an appointment or take some time off. "The way our culture is so interdependent, it makes it really hard," she said.

Some of the students or physicians Gold works with have found her services essential to unearthing the reasons for, and addressing, profoundly challenging circumstances, such as the inability to sleep. More than once, Gold has worked with an individual experiencing insomnia only to discover that it was caused by the loss of a patient weeks prior— but because the trauma took some time to affect them, they hadn't made the connection. In such cases, Gold prescribes light sleeping medication while providing counseling until the doctor is able to understand and address the reasons for their insomnia, and then hopefully discontinue the medicine. "If you keep all that inside it just sort of festers and causes both physical and psychological symptoms, because that's what trauma does," Gold said. "Understanding and making sense of the narrative is just very eye-opening and clarifying."

When incidents occur that are overtly traumatic—such as a staff suicide, or workplace violence—hospitals will sometimes call in experts from organizations such as the International Critical Incident Stress Foundation (ICISF) to help staff manage the trauma. Director of Education and Training Victor Welzant, who also supervises a response team of twenty individuals at Sheppard Pratt Health Care in Maryland, said that ideally, resilience training begins prior to a critical incident in order to develop habits, behaviors, and mindsets—such as exercise, proper nutrition, and gratitude practices—that are conducive to mental health. Then, once a crisis occurs, it's essential to do a careful assessment. "The first thing is not making any assumptions about who needs what, but to ask," said Welzant, adding that interventions can involve any combination of—ideally voluntary—group discussions, one-on-one counseling, peer support, and education about typical stress responses and behaviors to promote recovery. While mental health professionals are part of these interventions, peer-to-peer engagement is a key component of ICISF's approach. "There's something about knowing that the other person has sort of walked in those shoes," Welzant said. "A credibility that's really helpful."

Welzant finds the most successful interventions are the ones in which healthcare practitioners rediscover what makes their work meaningful. "People walk away from it reminded of why they're there in the first place," said Welzant, recalling a healthcare worker who'd experienced a great deal of both personal and work stress and who was subjected to a violent event in the emergency room. She was ready to quit when a peer supporter suggested that she take some time off and seek counseling through the hospital's employee assistance program (EAP) instead. The staff member did so, and eventually returned to work. "One of the things we always say is don't make a major life decision in the middle of a crisis," Welzant said.

Many hospitals and other healthcare providers pay into EAPs that offer private, protected mental health services—including therapy, substance abuse counseling, and resources to promote work-life balance—though their use may still necessitate disclosure to a medical licensing board. For Amy Tilley, a psychologist and clinical director of the Desert Star Addiction Recovery Center in Tucson, Arizona, EAPs have proved essential for both herself and her staff. She recalled a particularly challenging period several years prior when the center, which provides both outpatient and partial hospitalization services, lost three of its clients to suicide in three months. Tilley took a mental health day to recover, surrounded by the beauty and serenity of nine-thousand-foot Mt. Lemmon. But as she left, her boss called to inform her that a fourth patient had died—this time, due to a horseback riding accident. "I just started crying," Tilley said. "That was the hardest one because she had done incredibly well and had some really super-high hopes."

Tilley said that following each incident, she would sit down with her staff, and asked what they needed. Many of them took advantage of the mental health services available through the center's EAP. "Just allowing people to feel, and talk about it, and be present, was really helpful," Tilley said. Tilley and another staff member also attended the fourth woman's funeral, which allowed her to process her grief and find some closure. "It was such a powerful moment," she said.

Even prior to these incidents, Tilley had been regularly engaging in her own personal therapy through the center's EAP, which helped her to process these and other traumas. "It's been an incredibly good neutral outlet," said Tilley, who finds that gaining insight into her childhood, adolescence, and college years has helped her grasp how they shaped her present experiences and relationships. While Tilley initially felt angry with those who'd committed suicide, therapy helped her release those feelings, as well as the sadness that came afterward. And when another young man died two weeks into treatment from what was termed an accidental overdose, which hit her really hard, Tilley spent six months discussing the case in weekly meetings with her therapist. Finally, the therapist suggested that she reach out to the man who'd referred the patient—and she did so, visiting him in his office. "He started crying as soon as I walked in," Tilley said. The two of them sat there and cried for a while before this man showed her the death certificate—which, somehow, enabled her to move on. "That was all it took," Tilley said. "It was the simplest thing."

In addition to the stress, burnout, and suffering that medical professionals encounter in the workplace, they undoubtedly experience their own personal struggles, challenges, and heartbreak. How much more essential, then, that they have safe and nonpunitive access to the support they need, and, when necessary, take advantage of it? By watching for warning signs like emotional exhaustion, mood changes, cynicism, and disconnection from patients, clinicians can take the opportunity to receive help—and by doing so, rediscover the vitality within themselves, and their chosen career. Welzant advised that "the more you use professional help to build resilience, the more you can also improve your performance as a physician, as a nurse—and restore your sense of meaning, your sense of energy about your work, your excitement for it, and your passion."

6

Education, Creativity, and Growth

Our ideas can enslave or liberate us.

—SIR KEN ROBINSON

Innovators have been emerging in the past few decades to address the damaging aspects of medical culture and to improve physician wellness by changing medical curricula, developing resources, offering retreats, providing coaching sessions, and more. Most have been motivated by their own educational and professional experiences, while some have stepped up in response to student and clinician concerns. Many have been inspired by recent research into physician burnout, including the work of Liselotte Dyrbye and Colin West at the Mayo Clinic, and Tait Shanafelt, formerly of the Mayo Clinic, who became the chief wellness officer for Stanford Medicine.

The gold standard for measuring burnout is the Maslach Burnout Inventory (MBI)—named for Christina Maslach, who developed the measure in 1981 to assess three subscales: emotional exhaustion, depersonalization, and a decreased sense of personal accomplishment. After observing the impact of interns' distress on patients as a senior resident at the University of Washington, Shanafelt worked with Anthony Back on his research rotation to apply Maslach's measure to residents and analyze the impact of physician burnout on the quality of care. The resulting study, which found that 76 percent of responding residents met the criteria for burnout and that burnout was strongly associated with self-reported suboptimal patient care, drew widespread attention when it was published in 2002. Later, Shanafelt partnered with Dyrbye, West, and others to co-author numerous studies, both of the educational system and the profession at large, that demonstrated the impact of a clinician's environment on burnout, the high cost of physician turnover, and more.

Stuart Slavin, a pediatrician, was the dean of medical curriculum at St. Louis University (SLU) in Missouri when he came across Dyrbye's work on depression, burnout, and suicidal ideation among medical students—including the study of more than four thousand students at seven US medical schools, published in the *Annals of Internal Medicine* in 2008, in which roughly 49.6 percent of students reported burnout, while 11.2 percent had experienced suicidal ideation within the past year. As it turned out, that discovery changed the course of his career.

"Not Healthy in Many Respects"

By the time Slavin encountered Dyrbye's research he'd been working to create a nurturing and supportive environment at SLU for the past three or four years. Most of the students seemed to be doing well, and Slavin had a hard time believing that nearly a third of them could be depressed. But then a survey of students in all four years revealed that he was wrong. "They looked great at orientation, but in every year they were suffering greatly," Slavin said. "When I looked at that, the only conclusion I could come to was that we were doing this to them. And as curriculum dean, I felt responsible."

Slavin was determined to change the curriculum—something he was more easily able to do in his position than administrators in student affairs, who typically assume responsibility for student wellness. (Other medical schools had improved access to counseling services; provided education on the issues of burnout, depression, and suicide; and created student wellness committees, among other interventions.) First- and second-year medical students at SLU had identified the main reasons for their distress to be: 1) the sheer volume of information they were required to absorb; 2) the level of detail inherent in this information; and 3) the competition for grades. As a result, the Office of Curricular Affairs reduced the curriculum by 10 percent for the incoming class of 2013, worked with faculty members to limit the information load, and introduced a pass/fail grading system. Moreover, electives were shifted to provide a half-day of free time every two weeks, and five learning communities were established that allowed students to engage with faculty and explore shared interests. Changes implemented in the following years included a compulsory six-hour resilience and mindfulness program, social events, and changes to the human anatomy exams that led to higher scores when assessing the mean of student exams, reducing the fear of failure.

By many measures, these adaptations were a success. Evaluations of first- and second-year students at orientation and at the end of each year found that rates of depression, anxiety, and stress dropped significantly following the interventions. Additionally, the students' mean score on the Step 1 US Medical Licensing Examination rose and continued to outperform the national average. "We fall into this trap of thinking more is always better," said Slavin, recalling the common analogy that learning in medical school is like drinking water from a fire hose. For some doctors-in-training, this overload becomes an existential as well as an institutional threat as they encounter *medical uncertainty*, or what sociologist Renée Fox identifies as "incomplete or imperfect mastery of available knowledge" combined with "limitations in current medical knowledge," and the difficulty of distinguishing between the two. As Slavin noted, "depressed and anxious students don't learn very well, and if you're pushing them too hard, they can't hold onto the essential information." Still, not everyone appreciated the changes. In February 2017, the Liaison Committee on Medical Education (LCME)—the accrediting body for US medical schools—put SLU School of Medicine on probation for curriculum management and other issues. Not long after, despite protests from students, Slavin was dismissed. The school revamped its curriculum to meet LCME requirements and was cleared by the accrediting body in October 2018. "I don't know how [the committee] looked at what we were doing and came to the conclusions that they did," Slavin said.

For the past several years, Slavin has been the senior scholar for well-being at the Accreditation Council for Graduate Medical Education (ACGME), the accrediting body for all US graduate medical training (or residency) programs. There, he's worked with others to develop a suite of well-being resources called AWARE that includes a two-hour video workshop for program directors to discuss cognitive skills and strategies with students; an app that uses cognitive behavioral therapy through video scenarios and other methods; and podcasts aimed to address the mindsets of individual clinicians and residents. While Slavin recognizes that the toxic environment of residency programs must be addressed—something that ACGME attempts to do through its program accreditation requirements—he has found that residents' automatic thoughts and cognitive distortions can exacerbate the negativity of their experiences. "It's not coming up with a false optimism, it's just not being so distorted that you're always kind of beating up on yourself," he said. One of the app's video scenarios addresses being embarrassed when not knowing the answer on rounds—something every resident experiences. While Slavin acknowledged that the Socratic teaching method—which he considers ideal for the clinical setting because it probes and solidifies residents' knowledge while filling in the gaps—can turn into destructive "pimping" in the wrong hands, he said that students' mindsets also play a role. "If their knowledge gap is exposed, even if the intent wasn't there, they can still feel bad," he said. After presenting a talk to third-year medical students about mindsets including perfectionism, imposter syndrome, and viewing performance as identity, one young woman thanked Slavin, saying he'd given her a vocabulary for her thinking when she'd believed she was "just screwed up."

Oana Tomescu, an associate professor of clinical medicine at the University of Pennsylvania's Perelman School of Medicine, was inspired by the impact of her own residency there, from 2004 through 2007, to address burnout and well-being among doctors-in-training. "The mentality of my generation at the time was pretty much: residency is tough, it's hard, it's going to be the worst time of your life, and you should just put your head down and push through it," she said. "So not healthy in many respects." Students and residents were not encouraged to engage in self-care, and Tomescu didn't see a doctor or a dentist for seven years. When she eventually caught up on her pap smears, Tomescu learned she had cervical cancer, requiring a hysterectomy at age forty-one. Fortunately, the cancer was localized, and Tomescu hadn't been passionate about the idea of having children, but it brought home the importance of changing systemic and cultural barriers to self-care. "It's not enough to say to residents, 'Don't forget about your doctors' appointments,'" Tomescu said. "It's also important to create the ecosystem to allow for these cultural changes." At the University of Pennsylvania, residents are now given six half-days for wellness each year during which they can schedule dentist appointments, get haircuts, or attend to other needs. "It's really challenging, especially during training when there's very little autonomy over one's schedule," Tomescu said.

Tomescu, whose research now focuses on preventing burnout in medical training, advocates for systemic change to address the six factors that Maslach identified as causes of burnout: lack of autonomy, perceived unfairness, moral distress, an imbalance between reward and effort, lack of community, and an excessive workload. And she works with students and residents to address the cultural mindsets that lead to burnout—including workaholism, perfectionism, competitiveness, and imposter syndrome—partly by developing better coping skills through mindfulness, self-compassion, and other strategies. "No one has ever heard this term self-compassion, and there's so much science behind self-compassion," Tomescu said. Students at the University of Pennsylvania are known to exhibit what is called "Penn Face," a facade of perfectionism that hides the pressure they're actually experiencing. (Other schools have similar terms, such as Stanford's "Duck Syndrome," which compares students to ducks that appear calm on the surface but are paddling furiously beneath.) "My mission has been, since my own training, to change the culture of medicine to one that is much more emotionally intelligent," Tomescu said. "Health systems have to be compassionate, too."

Another innovator who's worked to bring emotional intelligence into medicine is Rachel Naomi Remen—who, at the request of medical students desiring instruction on the role of the heart and the soul in medicine at the University of California, San Francisco (UCSF), created a curriculum called "The Healer's Art." First offered at UCSF in 1991 as a student-initiated elective, the course grew exponentially, and is now available at more than seventy medical schools in the US and around the world. The curriculum aims to help students uncover and strengthen their values, their sense of calling, and their desire to serve through principles drawn from psychology, contemplative studies, the creative arts, and other methods.

Evangeline Andarsio, the director of the National Healer's Art Program, was about ten years into her private practice as an obstetrician and gynecologist in Ohio when she began feeling burned out. Andarsio loved her work and being with her patients. But once the professional liability crisis—which had a particularly grave impact on obstetrics—hit her state, and many of her colleagues began leaving the specialty, she began to do some soul-searching. A friend pointed her to Remen's book, *Kitchen Table Wisdom: Stories That Heal,* and eventually Andarsio found herself attending a workshop that Remen led for physicians in California focused on meaning, grief, and loss. Andarsio, who was grieving the loss of her mother with diabetes to multisystem organ failure at the time, found the workshop a transformative experience. "I reconnected with my calling," she said. Andarsio eventually started a group, based on Remen's model, for her medical community in 2004, followed by The Healer's Art program at Wright State University's Boonshoft School of Medicine two years later.

Andarsio said that The Healer's Art course is important because while medical school is focused on delivering large volumes of information, most people choose the profession for heartfelt reasons. "The human aspect of medicine is what really connects us to the meaning of our work," Andarsio said. "It's such a key piece to the healing of the patient. And I would dare say this: the healing of the healer." The Healer's Art, she said, creates a space where students have permission to bring their whole selves into the process of medicine and to integrate their values, priorities, and ethics. "It allows students to be who they are," she said. While The Healer's Art program has become increasingly popular in medical schools, its availability to other practitioners remains limited. Some organizations provide a nurse-focused version, "The Power of Nursing," while a handful of physician assistant and physical therapy programs also offer, or are planning to offer, The Healer's Art. Meanwhile, the University of Washington has an interprofessional program based on the curriculum.

Key aspects of The Healer's Art include discovering and nurturing one's wholeness; addressing grief and loss; embracing mystery and awe; and engaging in service as a way of life. "This course honors all faith traditions and also those with no faith tradition," said Andarsio, who has found it to be powerfully rooted in self-discovery and transformation. "We not only self-discover what's important to us, what our values and priorities are in medicine, and in how we want to be as physicians, but we also explore our life experiences." Thanks to the course, Andarsio said students have reported feeling more connected to patients and colleagues, while faculty are able to reconnect with their work and view students as humans again. For Andarsio, the workshop with Remen helped her to rediscover the mystery and awe in her work as an obstetrician, which she returned to for another fifteen years. "We can't lose our sense of wonder in what we do," said Andarsio, who said it was easy to get bogged down in the day-to-day tasks or experience a sense of numbness—even when performing such an awe-inspiring task as delivering babies. "We look for those nuggets of mystery throughout our day to maintain meaning in our work and give us that sense of aliveness," she said.

Since 2016, the University of New Mexico (UNM) School of Medicine has made The Healer's Art course a mandatory part of its roughly thirty curriculum hours pertaining to well-being. While some pushback occurred initially, 51.6 percent of students were open to enrolling after taking the course, a dramatic increase of 19.4 percent from those who would have done so prior to the experience (32.2 percent). Elizabeth Lawrence, the school's chief wellness officer and assistant dean of professional well-being, said her response to the remaining students who would have preferred that time for other activities is that "we're teaching skills and demonstrating our commitment to your well-being. And that's really important."

Lawrence said that UNM's approach is based on the Stanford Model of Professional Fulfillment, which recognizes the need to address three major areas: a culture of wellness, efficiency of practice, and personal resilience. In an effort to improve environmental factors, the school has implemented pass/fail grading, as well as "wise weeks" scheduled between intense courses that allow students time to decompress. Students spend all four years in a learning community called a "house"—sometimes compared to those in the Harry Potter novels—along with a faculty mentor, which builds community and allows junior and senior students to learn from each other. Meanwhile, a Learning Environment Office provides an avenue for students or residents to make confidential complaints about mistreatment.

To further address imbalances in the medical culture, Lawrence has partnered with others at the school and in the larger community to destigmatize mental health issues by hosting panels of physicians in recovery from substance abuse; publicizing personal support resources and counselors; and lobbying the medical board to change the language on New Mexico's licensing application. Now, rather than being asked about past physical injuries or diseases, impairments, or mental health issues, physicians are questioned about current impairments that would interfere with their ability to provide care. "That was a big success," Lawrence said. In addition, the school offers matriculating students and residents opt-out—rather than opt-in—wellness checks with a counselor, which has been embraced by more than three-quarters of both cohorts, she said. "By showing that's the normal, to have the appointment, I think we're sending a powerful message," Lawrence said. "And it's increased the use of our services quite a bit." Still, she recognizes that there's further to go in addressing medical student and resident burnout, including addressing systemic racism; finding ways to minimize the burden of the electronic medical record; and reducing the strain on faculty who are expected to increase clinical productivity while also teaching and mentoring students.

"Community Through the Arts"

Other innovators are exploring ways of incorporating the creative arts into medical education and practice. Research generally supports the efficacy of the arts in reducing stress and burnout: one 2014–2015 study published in the *Journal of General Internal Medicine* found that medical students exposed to literature, music, theater, and the visual arts—both as engaged participants and as spectators—demonstrated higher levels of empathy, tolerance for ambiguity, greater wisdom, and other positive qualities, while also experiencing significantly less burnout.

As a student at Rutgers Robert Wood Johnson Medical School in New Jersey, Daniel Marchalik initiated a literature and medicine elective to engage students in literary discussion, introspection, and narrative analysis. Later, after completing his residency and obtaining a Master of Arts in English literature, both at Georgetown University in Washington, DC, Marchalik created a four-year Literature and Medicine track there in 2013, which he now oversees as an associate professor of urology.

Participating students read eight to nine novels per year and then come together to discuss them; in 2020 they read Sally Rooney's *Normal People*, Jhumpa Lahiri's *The Interpreter of Maladies*; and Ocean Vuong's *On Earth We're Briefly Gorgeous*, among others. In addition, authors are brought in to meet with students, and students produce a capstone project in their final year. One student wrote an article about his regrets around being a kidney donor after reading Kazuo Ishiguro's *Never Let Me Go*, which he published in *The Washington Post*. Another created a program that trained first-year medical students to write obituaries for their cadavers in anatomy class by reaching out to and interviewing the donor's family members—now, a standard part of the course. "Even though none of these books are about medicine, they're all about medicine," Marchalik said of the novels. "That's just what we see every day. But it does give you a different window into how to process it or think about it."

Marchalik has conducted research studies among European and US urology residents, in addition to US palliative care providers. His findings show that for all of them, reading for pleasure was evidently protective against burnout. "It prevents depersonalization because it gives you the chance to step into someone else's shoes and imagine other worlds," said Marchalik, who believes that widespread burnout in urology is likely influenced by the cognitive and emotional burden of dealing with complex cancer patients combined with busy clinics and a heavy documentation burden. "And to give people complexity, to give them the benefit of the doubt and understand that they have their own issues and difficulties." Marchalik believes this impact is different than what somebody gains from watching television, because as a reader, one is required to use one's imagination rather than view another's creation. In addition, "there's a different cadence to reading than there is to watching a TV show, and I think that makes a really, really big difference," he said.

Marc Moss, a pulmonary critical care doctor, professor, and vice chair of clinical research for the department of medicine at the University of Colorado School of Medicine, has been heading a research lab that is exploring the impact of creative arts therapies on stress and job satisfaction among healthcare professionals. In 2020, the Colorado Resiliency Arts Lab (CORAL) launched four different modalities for clinicians to explore—including art therapy, dance movement, music therapy, and a writing workshop, in addition to a control group. While the twelve-week program was initially designed for those working in critical care, once the COVID-19 pandemic hit, the lab opened its doors to all healthcare workers in the Denver metropolitan area, realizing all had been deeply affected. Participants—mostly nurses, but also physical therapists, respiratory therapists, and physicians—met once a week for an hour and a half to engage in prescribed activities. "People love it," Moss said. "People like the sense of community and the safe space we give people to talk about some difficult things."

Moss, who by September 2020 had spent six months living in his basement for fear of infecting his family with COVID-19, said that healthcare workers have always had stressful and traumatic jobs. "It's not really a mental health issue, it's really more of an occupational health issue," he said, quoting from Walt Whitman and Louisa May Alcott, both of whom were nurses during the American Civil War, to prove his point. Yet Moss has found that the medical profession typically downplays the psychological strain of the work, and that stigma, bureaucracy, and a medical culture that values stoicism all contribute to burnout. "We're taught a lot in medical school to depersonalize; to not always view people as people," he said. "I think it's an okay defense mechanism, but I don't think it's an ideal mechanism."

While Moss acknowledges the systemic drivers of burnout and need for organizational interventions, he's come to believe that people needed a creative outlet to express their trauma in nonverbal ways. And the CORAL initiative has demonstrated that there's clearly an interest. While the pandemic limited the size of the program's four groups to ten, including an instructor, by September 2020, 36 people were participating and the program had a wait list of more than 150. Moss believes that part of its effectiveness lies not just in providing a creative outlet, but also in reducing the sense of isolation and loneliness that are common among healthcare workers—even when there isn't a pandemic. "It's another way to build a sense of community through the arts," he said.

For Joseph Schlesinger, an anesthesiologist, ICU doctor, and associate professor at Vanderbilt University School of Medicine in Nashville, Tennessee, music is not only a tool that can be used to engage clinicians and patients, but also an innovative intervention that can be applied in the hospital setting. Schlesinger, an accomplished jazz pianist who had studied music and sound in relation to neuroscience, partnered with Ruth Kleinpell, an associate dean at the Vanderbilt School of Nursing, to create a research project called Music in the ICU. Relying largely on a piano, painted in vibrant colors by a local artist, in addition to the occasional flute, cello, or violin, the program brought volunteers—mostly undergraduate students from the university's Blair School of Music—into the medical ICU several times a week to perform high-quality classical music for patients and staff. Often, they would wheel the piano into the rooms; other times, they would play from the hallway. Some patients declined—usually, when there was a football game on. But even those initially skeptical responded well. "Their affect would soften, and then the family members would get into all these stories" about the piano, Schlesinger said. "It was not uncommon to see tears of joy or comfort." He recalled one patient who'd been minimally responsive for his entire ten-day stay when a volunteer played at his family's request. The patient's physiology began to normalize—his heart rate slowed, and his low blood pressure came up—and then, he began to conduct a little bit with his right hand. "It was the most responsive he'd been to his environment since his hospitalization," Schlesinger said. "The family was tearful; we were awestruck."

Patients were not the only ones to benefit from the intervention. Schlesinger found that nurses would gather around, and residents would take a mini-break, to watch; many thanked him for the project. "It seemed to really help their mood and their sanity," Schlesinger said, adding that they chose classical music based on the literature showing that it had positive neurological effects, and live music to create a multisensory experience including richer sound, the visual component of a musician performing, and the music's tactile vibration. For clinicians working in the ICU, who are constantly exposed to beeping alarms and other jarring noises, Schlesinger believes such auditory interventions can have significant impact. He hopes that their implementation study will inspire other institutions to replicate and build on the program. "It's non-invasive, it's low-risk, potential high reward," Schlesinger said. "It would be great if we could think of sound exposure as being helpful or harmful. And how do we prescribe it."

Another creative endeavor that has been boosting well-being and resilience among nurses is Project Knitwell. Founded by Executive Director Carol Caparosa, the organization has been teaching hospital staff and patients in Washington, DC, to knit—beginning with simple projects such as a hat, a cowl-knit scarf, or fingerless gloves—before progressing, for those who are interested, to more advanced patterns. Caparosa was inspired to found the organization after her daughter was diagnosed with multiple congenital heart defects at just seven days old, and Caparosa spent much of her time at MedStar Georgetown University Hospital. She rediscovered knitting, which she'd once had an affinity for, while waiting for her daughter to come through multiple long surgeries. "I'd just knit and knit, and somehow I felt better," Caparosa said. "I felt like I was making something, even though I never finished anything."

After her daughter turned fifteen, Caparosa returned to Georgetown to "give back" and began working with mothers of pediatric cancer and transplant patients. Project Knitwell has since been in seven hospitals in addition to working with women who are struggling with homelessness or in prison. "Some mothers I worked with, they weren't even able to hold their baby for three weeks because the baby was so fragile," said Caparosa, who spent a good deal of time in the newborn ICU. "But they were able to knit a hat, and they could see the baby wearing a hat. So that's huge."

Despite the fact that the organization has been working in hospitals for ten-plus years and a research study found the knitting intervention had the ability to significantly reduce burnout and compassion fatigue among nurses, Caparosa said it's often difficult to engage nursing staff because they are often so busy while on duty and are reluctant to come in on days off. However, after Project Knitwell went virtual due to the pandemic, things changed. Caparosa found that the majority of their initial sign-ups were nurses—particularly from MedStar Georgetown University Hospital, where the offering was first promoted. Each nurse was assigned to a volunteer, and received live, one-on-one classes over video chat. "Everybody feels a sense of accomplishment, especially when they finish their project—but mostly, people talk about the calming effect," said Caparosa, citing Betsan Corkhill, a UK-based therapeutic knitting expert who's found the rhythmic motion of knitting to induce a form of meditation. "They've told us how much it's meant to them, and how they feel a little less stressed."

"Who Owns Your Joy?"

Another means that physicians and nurses have found to reduce stress and gain support is to engage in retreats or workshops for healthcare professionals that provide continuing education, a supportive environment, mindfulness training, and other benefits. Some focus on providing clinicians with the skills they need to address the emotional strain of their careers. Others address damaging mindsets, provide methods of navigating systemic challenges, or offer alternatives to the traditional medical model. Regardless, simply spending time with other clinicians in an inspired setting often provides the kind of connection, nourishment, and sense of well-being that many are seeking.

Kathy Stepien, a pediatrician in Juneau, Alaska, had longstanding involvement in community-building and wellness retreats when she decided to found the Institute for Physician Wellness in 2016 and began offering retreats in locations around the country—and even one in Baja California, Mexico. "I knew what I felt myself—the sense of isolation and also the recognition that the culture of medicine's not a healthy one," Stepien said. "And I knew that there were other physicians that were really struggling."

Stepien typically hosts at least three retreats per year for anywhere from eight to over one hundred physicians, though she tries to keep them on the smaller side to prevent them from feeling like a conference. "It's healing for physicians to be with other physicians because we understand the culture," she said. "What it's like to have that responsibility, and have the joys and the struggles and the self-sacrifice and everything that goes with medicine." The retreats offer continuing medical education classes on topics including finding permission for joy; secondary trauma; how to negotiate the inner critic and imposter syndrome; gender equity and other forms of microaggression and implicit bias; and more. In addition, small group discussions revolve around the interests of those in attendance, such as time management, loneliness, or finding work-life integration as a parent. "People talk about how it's changed their lives and they wish they'd experienced this earlier in their career," Stepien said.

Following repeated requests for consulting or mentoring, Stepien began to offer physician coaching—a role she was initially reluctant to assume but later embraced as studies provided convincing evidence that linked coaching to improved well-being. "It helps physicians develop skills so that they can be healthy and decrease emotional exhaustion," Stepien said. "Physicians can help other physicians develop those skills." She also teaches mindfulness-based stress reduction to healthcare professionals in all roles, and has found that the two overlap in many ways. "It's really about tapping into that sense of agency and becoming aware of how our beliefs play out for us," said Stepien, who often finds herself addressing negative thought patterns such as: "I'm stuck"; "It's all the fault of the electronic medical record"; or "I have student loans that I'll never be able to repay." While Stepien acknowledges that such beliefs are based on real organizational and structural issues, her hope is that by improving personal well-being, clinicians will recover enough to tackle those larger challenges more effectively. "One of the questions I ask is: 'Who owns your joy?'" she said. "Because I don't want an insurance company to own it, or the pandemic."

Over the years, Stepien has come to learn how profoundly physicians are struggling. "Healthcare professionals share with me how incredibly broken they feel," she said. "They may look okay on the outside, but on the inside there's a depth of suffering that is breathtaking." Stepien finds her role incredibly rewarding, as she's not only helping physicians, but also their patients, families, and communities. "I see this ripple effect," she said. Still, she said there remains a need for significant institutional reform around how healthcare is delivered in the US, including a universal healthcare plan for all Americans; a universal electronic medical record that is functional, effective, and efficient; sufficient time to attend to patients; and a structure that allows healthcare professionals to work at the highest level of their training. Particularly post-pandemic, Stepien said, a lot of "repair work" needs to happen "between frontline workers and the institutions, and what the expectations are for serving humanity, for serving our community."

Jan Landry, who worked as a hospice nurse and chaplain in California for more than thirty years, left the field in 2010 partly because she no longer felt aligned with the system's growing levels of regulation, bureaucracy, and repetitive paperwork. She did some mindfulness training and then began to teach mindfulness workshops—often, to healthcare providers disillusioned by the manner in which staffing issues were jeopardizing patient safety and quality of care. "Many of them get into the work because they really care and they want to make a difference," Landry said. "So that takes a deep toll on people's hearts and minds and creates a great stress."

Early on in her hospice career, Landry began partnering with a nurse colleague, Patricia Dunbar, after the two of them realized that while their skills and knowledge were helpful, the most effective healing happened through their presence. "This part of nursing doesn't really get talked about in a direct kind of way, but it's really the heart," said Landry, recalling a time when a patient's daughters had pointed out the manner in which a home health aide was bathing their mother with deep respect, as though anointing her. "There's something very holy when we're that present with somebody in their rawness, in their vulnerability, when things are falling apart." In the '80s, the duo held a handful of workshops for nurses related to this phenomenon before taking a long break. Around 2012, they began to offer workshops again through their organization, The Sacred Art of Nursing, which draws on the framework of mindfulness to help nurses take care of and support themselves.

The Sacred Art of Nursing's workshops and weekend retreats aim to bring nurses together as a community and help them to reestablish their relationships with themselves. "One of the things that happens when the outside demands are so big is that people can lose connection," Landry said. "That loss of connection with oneself is a huge stressor, because when we're disconnected, when we're unaware, then we become out of balance. So part of what we're trying to do is to help people find ways to come back home to their own experience." One way that Landry does this is through guided meditation and mindful check-ins, during which participants feel into their bodies, hearts, and minds to see where there's tension. "Learn to really pay attention to your own experience, to listen to it in a very kind way, without judgment," she said. "And then try to incorporate some self-care, and that becoming connected, into day-to-day life."

Often, Landry advises nurses to recognize when they can take a moment—such as when washing their hands—to be kind to themselves, regain a sense of presence, and prepare to connect to their next patient as a whole person. And when they get home, she encourages them to take time to process their feelings—whether positive or negative—rather than bypassing or overriding them. In her workshops, nurses practice setting boundaries through role-playing by acknowledging a concern, setting a limit, and redirecting. The result is something like: "I can see we're really short-staffed and you need somebody to work that extra shift tonight. I'm not able to do that. Is there a way I can help you to think about this?" Nurses need such practice, Landry said, "because our hearts care. But we end up betraying ourselves."

While there are systemic reasons for the stressful nature of the nursing environment, Landry said that these are things healthcare workers can do to protect themselves—including retaining an inner sense of unhurriedness, and remembering that life and death are mysterious and there are larger forces at play. She recalled one ICU nurse who described herself and her colleagues as being in a constant state of tension—bracing for the next event—even when things were slow. "It's hard to unwind from that unless you begin to recognize it," she said. "I know some nurses who carry a small rock in their pocket as a way to just say, 'Okay, I'm grounded to the earth. Here's my ground.'" Sometimes, she said, retired nurses are drawn to her workshops in a desire to process undigested stress and trauma. "Some of what we're doing is bearing witness, and it can begin to normalize," she said.

For Emily Piper, an oncology nurse in Colorado, attending retreats with cancer survivors has given her an opportunity to explore her own unaddressed feelings while viewing patients in a new light. For about five years, Piper has been on the medical team with Epic Experience, an organization that provides weeklong outdoor retreats to cancer survivors in the Colorado Rockies—some of whom have stage four cancer and are still undergoing treatment. She's attended two summer camps and one winter camp, and engages in all of the activities—such as whitewater rafting, horseback riding, and cross-country skiing. "I don't think survivors realize when they go to camp that maybe there are things they haven't processed, maybe they need to talk to somebody else," said Piper, who would often sit around evening bonfires and just listen, contributing when she felt inspired to do so or when campers asked for her perspective. "I get to camp and feel all of the same emotions of, yes this is amazing and fun but I maybe didn't process that patient I lost four months ago. I didn't have the time, now that I'm here and have a chance to breathe again and talk to people who know what I'm going through. It's just an amazing feeling of letting go and transformation." Piper said that she's cried at every camp she's attended, and returns to work feeling rejuvenated.

Many institutions value the importance of such time away—including the University of New Mexico, which has offered an annual writing retreat for healthcare professionals in Taos for more than two decades based on a recognition of the importance of reflecting on and writing about their experiences in medicine. Over the years, the retreat has evolved to include wellness activities such as optional yoga, movement, and dance sessions, as well as discussions of the Stanford Model and how to bring the feeling of the retreat back into daily life. "I think an opportunity to pause and to not have that pressure, and to build community and build connection, is so key for well-being," Lawrence said.

One unique approach is that of Pamela Wible, who leads retreats for those who've given up on adapting to the environment and are looking to establish an alternative. Wible, the physician advocate who's spent years researching physician suicides and who was herself suicidal for six weeks after becoming disgusted with "assembly-line, big box medicine," realized there were other options. She'd tried six jobs over ten years, and in every one, she'd felt her job description boiled down to "See as many patients as you can, churn them through, and just bring them back if they have another problem." Wible told her patients how she was feeling, and they agreed—so she created her own wellness center based on their recommendations, which opened in Eugene, Oregon, in 2005. "I've been super happy ever since," she said. "No more problems with my mental health."

Wible began leading retreats for physicians looking to launch an independent practice—many of whom had also become suicidal. She realized the extent of the issue after asking physicians at a business strategy retreat how many of them had lost a colleague to suicide. Everyone's hand went up. Next, she asked how many had been suicidal themselves, and only one hand went down. "The number one main reason for many people is either a huge level of disillusionment to the point that they end up suicidal," she said, "or sort of that slow progressive irritation from being in the wrong, hazardous working environment over time that will wear on your soul and make you feel like you're just going through the motions."

These days Wible holds retreats for individuals as well as groups of up to fifty people—though she's leaning toward more frequent, smaller retreats at various locations around the country. They still cover business strategy, but because she's gained such a reputation as a physician mental health advocate, many who attend have been suffering from occupationally induced mental health conditions. "People are coming to receive help and healing from the trauma of their medical training and being trapped in medical practices that are really crushing to their hearts and souls," said Wible, who would like to see physicians granted the same labor rights as others in terms of their mandated hours and breaks. "And so we end up having to spend half the retreat, at least the first day, helping everyone get quick, rapid healing and validation." From there, she discusses what physicians wrote on their personal statements when they first applied to medical school and then explores what their ideal clinic or working environment would look like and helps them take steps to realize that goal. Wible said that while medical students, nurse practitioners, and physician assistants have attended, the majority of her participants are doctors—even some in their seventies, who are looking to establish a practice more in line with their values before they retire. Around 90 percent of participants have taken steps to open their own clinics, she said.

Those who remain in the traditional medical model, meanwhile, must continue to find ways to navigate the challenges inherent in the system—through personal self-care practices, mindfulness, and other tools—while advocating for institutional reform. Although there have been some encouraging shifts in approaches to medical education and training based on the Stanford Model, The Healer's Art, and other innovations, these have not been enough to stem widespread depression and burnout among healthcare workers, both in the educational system and in healthcare at large. As a result, clinicians are largely left to find their own ways of dealing with the mental, emotional, and physical strain. For some, like Wible, that means opening their own practice. For others, it can mean leaving the profession altogether. Many develop unique and creative means to retain their sense of empathy and compassion and to establish a greater sense of harmony between their work and the rest of their lives.

Reducing Empathic Strain through Balance, Compassion, and Joy

Not even one's own pain weighs so heavy as the pain one feels with someone, for someone.

—MILAN KUNDERA

After losing her mother to breast cancer when she was in her early twenties, Caroline Cárdenas was inspired to become an oncology nurse. "The empathy and the compassion that were spilling over in my heart made me want to come to the side of patients and their families who were experiencing that," said Cárdenas, who worked in Florida, New York, and California in specialties including radiation oncology, breast medical oncology, and head and neck cancer. Eventually, while working full-time at an infusion center in San Diego and studying for her master's degree, Cárdenas experienced full-on compassion fatigue and burnout. She was juggling numerous responsibilities—sometimes handling four or five patients at once; managing numerous cytotoxic chemotherapy agents;

establishing trust with patients who were sometimes receiving chemotherapy for the first time; adhering to strict safety protocols; and working against the clock, amid other challenges. Under the circumstances, Cárdenas didn't feel able to care for her patients the way she wanted to. "A caring heart requires an open heart, which requires an empathetic heart, which requires a compassionate heart," she said. "It just got to a point where it was far too much." While Cárdenas found ways to enhance her sense of joy and satisfaction through playful activity, she eventually left the position, and—after getting married, having a daughter, and entering her final year of doctoral coursework at Meridian University— retired from nursing. As a play psychology researcher, Cárdenas's PhD dissertation focuses on how play impacts helping professionals experiencing compassion fatigue.

While empathy and compassion inspire many healthcare workers to pursue their role in the first place, it can be difficult to maintain a compassionate stance in a system that emphasizes profit and time management—often at the expense of patient care. In addition, clinicians must find ways to process and manage empathic strain as they confront violent traumas, dying patients, and grieving family members. For many, their ability to do so is greatly impacted by whether or not they can find balance between work responsibilities and other aspects of their lives, connect with their own family, and care for their own health. While empathy can be a powerful motivating force, it can also leave clinicians feeling overwhelmed, or cause them to shut down—an ineffective coping mechanism that harms their well-being as well as that of their patients. For each individual, finding ways to conceptualize and process their feelings—while remaining compassionately engaged with patients, and themselves—is a journey.

"The Armor Thing's Not Working"

Researchers and psychologists have long analyzed the role of compassion in healthcare, while many educational programs are just beginning to discuss its significance for aspiring clinicians. Traditionally, healthcare workers have been taught to maintain some emotional distance from patients in order to display professional capability and protect their mental health. But increasingly, clinicians are beginning to embrace the benefits of staying connected, while drawing on tools such as mindfulness and meditation to enhance compassion for themselves and their patients. While displaying emotion in healthcare is still a questionable practice for many, repressed feelings often find a way of surfacing, regardless—and not always in the healthiest ways.

Meeta Shah, an assistant professor of emergency medicine at Rush Medical College in Chicago who's been an attending physician for about twelve years, said that traumatic situations—including burn victims, cardiac arrests, sexual assault victims, or child abuse patients—were initially very difficult to handle. "The first time you ever see something like that it really imprints you," she said. Over time, Shah, who has a heart-shaped face and gentle manner, began compartmentalizing her feelings so that she could move on to the next patient. And for the most part, it worked—although sometimes it resulted in her having a shorter fuse or a sense of stress that seemed unrelated. But as time went on, Shah began having flashbacks to earlier, similar cases in which she hadn't dealt with her emotions. Once, after resuscitating a young woman, Shah recalled a similar situation in the past and abruptly left the room to cry. "It forced me to feel those feelings again," she said.

Now, when Shah experiences personal losses, such as the death of her grandparents, tears don't come as easily as they did before. "It starts to seep into other parts of your life when you become compartmentalized like that," she said. But since Shah became a mother—she has two young children—she's begun to feel things more deeply again, to care about the social aspects of her patients' lives, and about people in general. "I think that's a good thing," she said. "I was avoidant before. I probably still am to a degree, but I'm trying to break that cycle."

In 1992, Carla Joinson coined the term *compassion fatigue* to describe a "loss of the ability to nurture" among some nurses in the emergency department due to stressors that included long work hours, complex patient needs, and emotional distress. Merriam-Webster defines the term in a medical sense as "the physical and mental exhaustion and emotional withdrawal experienced by those who care for sick or traumatized people over an extended period of time." It is often used interchangeably with *secondary traumatic stress*, which refers to the indirect trauma experienced by those who are exposed to the graphic details of others' traumatic experiences.

But in recent years, this terminology has been changing. Françoise Mathieu, a compassion fatigue specialist and co-executive director of TEND, an Ontario, Canada-based organization offering resources and training for those in high-stress, trauma-exposed workplaces, said that experts in the field are retiring *compassion fatigue* in favor of *empathic strain*. The new term doesn't necessarily involve trauma, and differentiates *empathy*—the ability to recognize, understand, and share the thoughts and feelings of another—from *compassion*, which involves a motivation to help and often results in action. As Stephen Trzeciak and Anthony Mazzarelli state in their book, *Compassionomics: The Revolutionary Scientific Evidence That Caring Makes a Difference*, which explores the vast impact of compassion on patients' health, "empathy *hurts*, but compassion *heals*. Accordingly, the key distinction here is that empathy is *feeling*, compassion is *action*."

Oana Tomescu, the associate professor of clinical medicine at the University of Pennsylvania, said that in her experience, the best way to prevent empathy fatigue is to learn and practice compassion strategies for oneself as well as others. "Compassion doesn't stop at empathy—you feel another's suffering, there's an internal urge to alleviate suffering, and an action of some kind that follows," she said. "That action could be complete silence and sitting present with someone else's pain and just creating that space. It could be doing a lovingkindness type of meditation, or breathing in someone's suffering, and breathing out kindness or love or wishing them well. It could be a hand on someone else's hand." Research has shown that compassionate action improves physiological and emotional outcomes for patients, while protecting providers against burnout. "You're human—if you stop feeling emotions, that's not good," Tomescu said, pointing out that depersonalization is a key indicator of burnout. Rather, Tomescu teaches students mindfulness practices to stay better connected to themselves and their patients and engages in a personal sitting meditation most mornings.

For Aseem Desai, a cardiologist specializing in heart rhythm disorders in southern California, lovingkindness meditation and other compassion-focused practices are part of what helped him to recover from a period of burnout that impacted his health to the point where he took time off to rebalance his life. "I started developing these different tools," Desai said. "Not only to help myself, but also to reconnect to other people, to reconnect to my patients, to reconnect to why I went into medicine, my colleagues, my family." In addition to exercising, improving his nutrition, and spending time in nature, Desai found mindfulness to be key. He attended a meditation retreat, followed by the 2017 American Conference on Physician Health in San Francisco, during which one of the speakers led the audience of several hundred in a lovingkindness meditation. Now Desai, who's Christian, engages in some spiritual practice each morning, meditates, goes for a run, and spends time with his family before heading to work. And as he traverses the parking lot from his office to the hospital to perform a surgery, he'll stop to meditate in his car for five minutes. "It's made a world of difference," Desai said. "And people notice the change. I mean, they can see it in terms of me being grounded, being calm."

Mathieu said that some common causes of empathic strain for healthcare workers include having a large number of similar cases—a diabetes educator who sees hundreds of patients with the same chronic challenges, for example—as well as patients who have personality disorders or other difficult situations. Rather than maintaining distance from patients, however, she advocates exploring other tools. "People feel that by creating barriers that they are protecting themselves, and I would disagree with that," Mathieu said. "The more you feel, the more you can also pause and reset yourself—but we know that the armor thing's not working." Often, she said, people can notice early signs of empathic strain such as insomnia or other somatic symptoms, and excessive use of numbing agents such as Netflix, substances, or compulsive shopping or eating. Worsening symptoms include irritability—often with family members; social withdrawal; and a loss of humor or overuse of dark humor. Mathieu said that by identifying individual warning signs, healthcare workers can address the issue early on. She recommends micro-skills such as a three-minute reset in which the first minute is spent looking around and naming five things one can see; the second on feeling into the body; and the third focusing on the breath. Another approach is taking a media audit to prevent "doomscrolling" by limiting online activity. "Protect your mornings and protect your evenings," Mathieu said. "I work in a high-stress, trauma-exposed environment, and those strategies really work." Still, she noted that empathic strain is influenced by a wide variety of other factors, including working conditions, personal vulnerability, and work-related traumatic grief and loss.

Maria Marzella Mantione, a clinical professor of community pharmacy practice at St. John's University in New York, would like to see compassion recognized and rewarded by healthcare corporations and administrators and believes that to do so would help stem high levels of burnout among community pharmacists. Many suffer moral distress when unable to provide high-quality patient care due to constant pressure to meet metrics in areas including immunizations, medication therapy management, and adherence outreach calls, she said. "It's the constant pressure to do more with less," she said, pointing out that community pharmacies have been experiencing widespread corporatization through companies such as CVS and Walgreens even earlier than many hospital conglomerates. A pharmacist could be helping someone just discharged from the hospital after a heart attack who's beginning multiple complex medications, while right behind them is a person purchasing vitamins. Meanwhile, many patients see pharmacists as customer service providers and don't understand when they need to take time to check with prescribers or inform them that their insurance has raised their copay. "Reward people for compassion, not volume," said Mantione, who's seen multiple pharmacists lose their jobs despite several decades of service because they're not as fast. "Helping shouldn't be detrimental to your performance evaluation. Helping should be the root of your performance evaluation."

Many patient advocates agree. In *Compassionomics*, Trzeciak and Mazzarelli outlined numerous studies finding that compassion displayed by healthcare providers had a measurably positive impact on patients' physiology, perception of pain, functional impairment, endocrine function, wound healing, immunity, and more. In one dramatic example, a doctor named Edward Viner credited the caring some nurses displayed when assisting him as a thirty-four-year-old, ventilated patient suffering from septic shock—rather than their medical acumen—for his recovery. One healthcare lawyer who was touched by the humane approach of his care providers when undergoing treatment for lung cancer founded the Boston-based Schwartz Center for Compassionate Healthcare in 1995; ever since, the organization has been working to develop and encourage compassion in medicine by training caregivers to engage with patients in a manner that affirms the humanity of both. The center launched Schwartz Rounds to provide healthcare workers with a forum to discuss the social and emotional issues of patient care, and they're now offered at hundreds of hospitals and other healthcare organizations around the world. Those who participate report improved teamwork and communication, lower rates of stress and isolation, and greater feelings of compassion toward patients.

Director of Programs Stephanie Adler Yuan said that rounds are an hour long and begin with three or four panelists from different disciplines offering stories about caring for a patient or family, which serves as a springboard for those participating to discuss their own experiences. "They reconnect people to why they do this work," Yuan said. "They allow you to sort of show who you are and what matters to you to your colleagues, and to see that in them as well." Yuan has attended Schwartz Rounds in an auditorium with hundreds of people, and in a small back room with ten attendees, and has found that "they were talking about the same thing." She appreciates the manner in which Schwartz Rounds— which include security guards, phlebotomists, and any other professionals who might interact with a patient—break down barriers and center marginalized voices, while also enabling leadership to display vulnerability. Once, Yuan attended Schwartz Rounds at a hospital serving a largely

Chinese community in which one of the panelists, an interpreter, said that every conversation she interpreted went into her ears, through her heart, and out her mouth. "When else does anyone else have a chance to say or hear this?" Yuan said. "And they'll be changed as a result."

During the pandemic, the Schwartz Center partnered with a psychologist from the National Center for PTSD to guide the implementation of trauma-informed Schwartz Rounds, both in person and on virtual platforms, to support the recovery of those experiencing trauma. Meanwhile, unit-based Schwartz Rounds allow organizations to bring the program into units, often at the request of a nursing manager, to address the needs of a specific group, while a new program called Stress First Aid provides organizations and staff with tools to recognize and address psychological stress before it becomes acute.

Still, Yuan recognized that Schwartz Rounds are just one method of addressing the suffering of healthcare workers amid widespread systemic and institutional challenges. Sometimes, healthcare systems will reach out to her hoping for a silver bullet, and she has to tell them that Schwartz Rounds are something to commit to over time. While the program will change an organization's culture and relationship with its staff, Yuan said, it needs to be part of a much broader effort to build trust. "It's just one piece of a real leadership commitment to systems change," she said. "Because honestly, that's what healthcare staff are really suffering from: trying to provide compassionate care within so many systemic challenges."

"It's about a Balanced Life"

Manoj Jain, an infectious disease physician in Memphis, Tennessee, had always maintained a challenging schedule. But after the COVID-19 pandemic hit, his responsibilities increased dramatically. In addition to seeing patients in the ICU and providing telemedicine, Jain served as an advisor to the mayor of Memphis, spending several hours a day on the phone and in meetings with policymakers. "It really feels like a war," said Jain, who worked from around 6:00 a.m. until midnight every day, watched his colleagues fall ill, and saw otherwise healthy patients come into the hospital starving for oxygen. "Each day something's happening, you're restrategizing, and that's what it feels like for us who are on the front lines." Meanwhile, Jain spent significantly less time with his wife, also a physician. And his daughter's wedding, which had been planned for seven hundred people on Memorial Day weekend, was reduced to just the bride's and groom's families and a priest.

Jain, who regularly meditates before bed, said that skills he developed around meditation and mindfulness helped him stay balanced, in addition to exercise and a plant-based diet. "I remember this level of stress only during my medical school years and during residency," he said. "It's very easy to spiral into a state of depression, almost resigned to the fact that we're doomed." While Jain was exposed to the concept of meditation as a child, when he would watch his grandmother rise at 4:30 a.m. every morning in India, it wasn't until adulthood that he became interested in the scientific basis for mindfulness. Now, he encourages his patients to engage in the practice, as well as the students he teaches at the University of Tennessee Health Science Center College of Medicine and Emory University's Rollins School of Public Health. The pandemic "will be an opportunity for us to reevaluate how we deal with our mental well-being, our emotional well-being," Jain said. Based on his research and experiences around mindfulness, Jain looks at happiness less as joy or pleasure than a sense of serenity, equanimity, and contentment. "A gift, or a piece of chocolate, or some ice cream, or a good movie—yes, it may give us joy and pleasure," he said. "But to achieve that level of equanimity, that lasting happiness that one talks about, that will come with the mindfulness, with that awareness."

While the COVID-19 pandemic imposed a series of unique circumstances for healthcare workers, maintaining work-life balance has been a longstanding concern for those facing ongoing hurdles such as extensive documentation requirements, widespread and uncoordinated quality metrics, and an inefficient electronic health record. Particularly for female clinicians, work-life balance can be uniquely challenging due to the dual demands of work and family, contributing to the higher rate of burnout reported by women physicians when compared to men. Despite the fact that there is a strong business case for making systemic changes to prevent burnout and related turnover (which costs US health systems an estimated $17 billion for physicians and $14 billion for nurses every year) clinicians often find themselves embedded in workplaces that are negatively impacting their health and relationships—at which point it may be in their best interest to leave. "I really think that ethically there are also times where it's time to go, to move to another institution, to take a break from a field," Mathieu said. "And I think we need to be able to say that." Surveys show that millennial physicians place a high value on work-life balance, reflected by the increasing trend of choosing high-paying specialties with more controllable hours such as dermatology that allow them to pay off student debt and reduce the strain on personal lives. Meanwhile, the majority of female physicians name work-life balance as their top concern, ahead of compensation, gender equality, and other issues.

Lara Bickford, a personable emergency physician in Portland, Oregon, chose the specialty, in part, for its more manageable hours—due to the stressful nature of the work, emergency doctors typically work less than 130 hours per month. As the mother of three small boys, Bickford has found that working for Northwest Permanente, in a pool of some eighty-five emergency physicians serving Kaiser Permanente hospitals, provides her with much-needed flexibility: She trades one of her two monthly overnight shifts for a less lucrative daytime alternative, leaving her with less income, but just one draining overnight shift per month. "Everyone understands that there's life outside of work," Bickford said of her group. "We kind of have each other's backs."

Bickford doesn't take on too many additional obligations such as committees or extra shifts in order to spend time with her family. And when someone makes a request that will overextend her, she's learned to say no—such as when her boss asked that she switch an overnight shift from home, managing facility transfers by telephone, for an in-hospital shift to cover for an injured colleague. There was a back-up system in place, and Bickford, who'd been juggling multiple duties during the pandemic with her children at home, requested it be used instead. "I felt so guilty," Bickford said. "But then I thought about it more, and thought: I'm super stressed out, I'm spread super thin right now, trying to do all this. And I need to say no."

Bickford said that she aims, within her schedule, to be able to exercise every day and have at least one meal with her family—whether that's breakfast, lunch, or dinner. When she gets overextended and that doesn't happen, Bickford finds she becomes more exhausted and less empathetic. "The empathy goes first," said Bickford, who reminds herself on her short drive to work why she cares for her patients, and that she wants to make an extra effort to stay connected. "There's a way of just making the patient feel like you're glad that they're there, and making them less worried about what's going on." Bickford also finishes her charting at the end of each shift—facilitated by the fact that Kaiser provides scribes who enter essential information, leaving her to wrap things up. Typically, physicians spend close to six hours charting per shift, including ninety minutes of after-hours "pajama time" finishing up their records. "That, for me, is huge," Bickford said of the scribes. "I spend more time with my patients, and I get out on time."

Nidhi Kukreja, a pediatrician in Chicago, said that it was only after leaving full-time work after five or six years to be home with her two young children that she realized how imbalanced she'd become. "There was this huge release, and this whole other side of life that I hadn't even realized I was missing," said Kukreja, who has sparkling brown eyes and an easy laugh. After a few years, she returned to practice part-time at a clinic in a predominantly Latino neighborhood on the southwest side of Chicago. Initially, she was overwhelmed by the emotional strain—such as patients who'd attempted suicide—in addition to the workload, partly because some 85 percent of their patients were on Medicaid, making it harder to secure referrals to specialists or early childhood interventionists. "I started meditating, and I talked to a couple of therapists and a career coach," said Kukreja, who also exercises regularly and introduced five minutes of mindfulness into weekly staff meetings. "I started to see that a lot of people were in the same boat, especially a lot of female physicians."

Kukreja realized that she didn't sleep well after staying up late to chart, so she stopped working at night. "I set up boundaries for myself, and it made a huge difference," she said. "I even changed my schedule so that I could try to do notes at work the next morning and then start seeing patients a little later. Because I don't like to leave work undone, even if it's notes, because I'm worried I'll forget something." Over time, Kukreja has become more comfortable with being a sounding board for patients with mental illness rather than simply prescribing medications. Recently, she'd spent an hour and a half on a video call with a patient on her day off. "You really have an impact and it's a nice thing," she said. "It takes time, though—it takes a lot of time."

While balancing between work and family is particularly hard for women, others also face this challenge. Arun Saini, a pediatrician at Texas Children's Hospital and assistant professor at the Baylor College of Medicine in Houston, has also found that his work-life balance has changed over time—along with his priorities. After completing his fellowship in pediatric critical care, Saini came out "all guns blazing" at his former institution, working a hundred hours a week or more to conduct and publish research and engage in multi-institutional projects in addition to his clinical duties. "I was already starting to be recognized as an important part of the team, and I felt like I was needed," Saini said. But in recent years—since his wife, a pediatric neurologist, lost her sister to breast cancer, they moved to a new city, and he had his second child—Saini has retrained his focus on his family.

These days, Saini works around fifty-five or sixty hours a week, and finds a sense of purpose in being of service to patients and their families. "That's the part that keeps me grounded," Saini said, recalling the recipient of a long-awaited lung transplant who didn't do well. "We see patients and families in their most vulnerable states, so when I see their struggles, I feel like, 'Oh, my struggles are just made up.'" When Saini realizes that he can no longer help a child, he'll shift his purpose to helping that child's family move through a difficult time. "The family really appreciates and remembers anybody who got involved," he said. "They remember everybody who ever entered that room." Still, Saini can think of several instances in which he was unable to extend himself in that manner due to exhaustion. "I didn't have it in me," he said. "Part of that is that we go through phases where you have to spend more time with [your own] family."

Finding the right work-life balance, preventing burnout, and building happiness often requires conscious effort. In his work, Alphonsus Obayuwana, a retired OB-GYN in Ohio who spent twenty-five years in teaching and faculty appointments, has developed a "mathematics of happiness" that he outlines in his book: *The Five Sources of Human Hope: Mirror of Our Humanity.* "I have delivered over four thousand babies, and every baby I've delivered came out unhappy," said Obayuwana, who was inspired to study human hope and happiness after encountering severely depressed psychiatric patients during his third year of medical school. "And it looks like for the rest of our lives we are in pursuit of happiness. As an obstetrician, that's the way I see it."

Being happy, Obayuwana found, requires identifying and supporting the five sources of hope in people's lives: Intrinsic assets, such as personal courage, ego strength, and self-esteem; human family assets, such as love and empathy from family and friends; economic assets, which refers to one's degree of economic contentment and sense of material sufficiency; educational assets; and spiritual assets. "If you don't realize these five important areas and you're just zeroing in on one of them, and you are overwhelmed by it, that's where the burnout comes from," said Obayuwana, who never experienced burnout despite a multi-decade career in a specialty that sees some of the highest rates of burnout in medicine. "These five areas, I made sure to pay attention to them, and that is the key for keeping yourself grounded and having a sense of satisfaction."

For Obayuwana, this meant taking small actions every day to support these areas of his life, no matter how busy he might be at work. To boost his educational assets, he made a conscious effort to learn something new every day and stay abreast of developments in his field. As a Catholic, he would increase his spiritual assets by taking a moment to make the sign of the cross; say a Hail Mary, Our Father, or the whole rosary when possible; or pray at a chapel on the way home from work. "Do something every day to pay attention to your soul," said Obayuwana, who is devoting the rest of his life to teaching the mathematics of happiness through his company, the Triple-H Project. "You just cannot get one thing and just drive that through and then forget other things. It's about a balanced life."

Moving the Dial

For many healthcare workers, finding a form of expression, or a means to increase their sense of joy and happiness, can be crucial when faced with empathic strain or burnout. About three or four years into her nursing career, Cárdenas—who had begun experiencing burnout and empathic strain while working at Memorial Sloan Kettering Cancer Center in New York—came across a man in Central Park who was playing the bongos and had laid out Hula-Hoops for passersby. Cárdenas stopped to watch, and was struck by the manner in which complete strangers responded to the phenomenon. "They were congregating and swinging this plastic circle around their body, and they would bring their arms up and erupt in joy," Cárdenas said. "So it was really simple, but it was powerful." The man convinced Cárdenas to try it—with her graceful stature, it came easily, and she stayed for three hours. That weekend, she bought her first Hula-Hoop and began using it in parks around New York. "I realized that it was changing me," she said. "I felt more alive, and I felt more joyful." When interacting with patients, Cárdenas noticed a new sense of joy, peace, and groundedness—"as if I had already tended to my joy and I had an abundance to offer."

Later, when she was experiencing even more stress in San Diego, Cárdenas would rush home from work, grab her Hula-Hoop and music, and cross the street to Windansea Beach, where she'd dance in circles on a rock, her layered hair swirling about her, as the sun was setting above the surfers in the ocean. "I was experiencing joy and it was sustaining me," said Cárdenas, who soon became known as "The Hula-Hoop Girl." After attending a boot camp in Santa Cruz to learn different hula-hooping techniques, she decided to write her master's thesis on hoop dancing as a means to prevent burnout and compassion fatigue among nurses, and it was published in the *Journal of Emergency Nursing* in 2014. Cárdenas began offering Hula-Hoop classes to nurses and also produced an annual, week-long Hula-Hoop retreat in Hawaii—something she continued, in addition to her studies and her clinical work, for around seven years. "What I witnessed was incredible," she said. "People were actually feeling empowered and believing in themselves and making big life choices." Cárdenas was inspired to pursue her doctorate in psychology and to write her dissertation on play—and its impact on helping professionals experiencing compassion fatigue. "It's a sacred experience," said Cárdenas, who has found a sense of absorption and freedom from time when hoop dancing that is comparable to meditation. "It's a place in which we discover who we are."

Another oncology nurse and nurse practitioner, Carolyn Phillips, was also inspired to seek out a form of expression and release after burnout and numbness set in. After nearly fifteen years working in both inpatient and outpatient settings, Phillips was studying burnout at a community cancer center in New Mexico when she began to discover the emotional roots of her own fatigue. "I started writing about patients I had cared for, who I was still carrying with me," Phillips said. "And that was okay, but I was still completely numb." Writing the stories down made Phillips aware of how many people she hadn't grieved, but it didn't quite "move the dial on that emotional feeling." So Phillips, who was also a musician, had her wife—as well as another, less familiar musician—put the experience to music. "The second I heard my story in music I felt the emotion," Phillips said. "And I cried like I hadn't cried in years."

The experience made Phillips curious as to whether other clinicians would react similarly. She recruited seven oncology and palliative care nurses from her former clinic to participate in a seven week-long workshop in Santa Fe, a pilot program during which they wrote their stories and read them aloud to each other. They learned to support each other in their emotions, and to not feel shame about having been personally affected. "Because I think there is shame," Phillips said. "We're taught to have strong boundaries, and that's how you do your work is you have to have strong professional boundaries, but that denies our human connection." For the final week, Phillips paired the nurses with musicians who set their stories to music, and both the stories and music were shared at a performance that was opened up to whomever they wanted to invite—close friends, family members, and colleagues.

Inspired, Phillips went back to school and obtained her doctorate and began researching how to work within systems to help healthcare professionals take care of themselves. Her nonprofit based on the pilot program—Songs for the Soul in Austin, Texas—offers programs, information, and support to professional caregivers, including workshops and retreats that pair nurses with songwriters. The workshops also teach participants to tune into their emotions through a body scan, as well as different meditation, mindfulness, and self-compassion tools—something Phillips considers essential for caregivers who are taught to put others before themselves. "For each person it's different," she said, in terms of what works. "For some people it's church; for some people it's nature; for some people it's family. Whatever it is that rejuvenates you."

For many, storytelling provides a mean of reconnecting to their patients, their colleagues, and themselves—providing what is perhaps the most widespread avenue in which healthcare workers have found a voice and form of expression. Since Rita Charon pioneered the first narrative medicine program at Columbia University in 2000, numerous programs have sprung up at medical schools around the country, including Oregon Health & Science University, the University of Southern California, and Temple University in Philadelphia.

Michael Vitez, a Pulitzer Prize–winning journalist who heads the Narrative Medicine Program at Temple University's Lewis Katz School of Medicine, said he was inspired to start building the program from scratch in 2016 because he "believed in the power of stories to heal and inspire and bring people together." He'd written numerous healthcare-related narratives during his thirty years on staff at *The Philadelphia Inquirer* and subscribed to the philosophy that sharing stories could improve trust and engagement with patients, enhance satisfaction in one's work, lead to better outcomes and patient care, and serve as a tool for physicians when advocating for their profession and their patients. Vitez, who speaks with a sense of palpable excitement about his efforts, worked with an assistant director, faculty member Naomi Rosenburg, and an associate dean to develop a variety of curricular and extracurricular offerings, including electives; workshops for residents; a formal certificate program (which may expand into a master's program); a literary magazine; and Story Slams.

Vitez holds multiple workshops in seven residency programs throughout the year. Residents begin with a short reading, usually a poem or short story unrelated to medicine—first to themselves and then out loud—and then discuss their insights; what they did or didn't like; and how it made them feel. They're then given a writing prompt, seven minutes to write, and the opportunity to share what they've written. "Extraordinary things can come out in seven minutes," said Vitez, who's found that roughly a third of residents are immensely grateful for the workshops, a third are skeptical but learn to love them, and a third don't really come around. "It just gets them seeing the world in stories, it gets them seeing their patients more completely," he said.

Story Slams, meanwhile, involve students, doctors, nurses, social workers, and anyone else who wants to participate. "It's really broad and inclusive and wonderful," said Vitez, who said that hierarchies are broken down, and he's watched the grill cook from the lobby of the medical school take the stage right before a big shot. "They tell stories about their own vulnerabilities, their own fears, mistakes they made, doubts they had, great surprises, things that happened, and it really just underscores for all of them why they got into medicine, the richness of medicine, the challenge of medicine." More experienced physicians tend to share stories about things they regretted earlier in their careers that made them better doctors, but weighed on them, while students often write about first experiences, such as watching someone die in the trauma bay, he said. "Everyone is lifted, both the storyteller and the story listeners."

Elizabeth Métraux, the founder and CEO of Women Writers in Medicine, has also found storytelling to have an uplifting impact on clinicians. In her former role as director of communications for workforce diversity at the National Institute of Health, Métraux conducted a multiyear research study across the country, interviewing individuals at all stages of their careers to understand drivers of burnout, particularly in relation to women and people of color. She found that when asked about what drove burnout, people offered a variety of answers. But when asked what drove fulfillment, she only got one: connection—whether to peers, patients, or purpose. "The natural follow-up is: Okay, how do we create connection?" Métraux said. "There's this profound need to tell our stories and to bring our whole selves into our work. And I saw that much more acutely with women and people of color."

In her current role, Métraux works with hundreds of women and organizations to obtain funding, publish research, and tell their stories. Through United Health Group in Austin, Métraux runs about four or five weekly sessions across the country in which one hundred to two hundred healthcare professionals gather for a guided discussion on topics such as community building or the power of stories. These are followed by virtual "huddles," in which healthcare workers of all stripes tell stories—including doctors, CEOs, nurse practitioners, and office staff. Sometimes, people share stories from the week prior. Once, those involved decided to share love stories—such as how they met their spouse or partner, or the one that got away—and the CEO of the health facility told how he'd married his seventh-grade sweetheart. "Here we are in the midst of this pandemic and a lot of these providers are so overwhelmed, and they wanted to tell love stories," Métraux said. "And I thought: Okay, well that's what we're going to do."

Others began drawing on narrative techniques to support clinicians during the COVID-19 pandemic. Meredith Mealer, the associate professor at the University of Colorado Anschutz Medical Campus, developed a narrative expressive writing program, which the American Nurses Foundation launched in May 2020 as part of its National Well-Being Initiative. Participating healthcare workers engaged in five weekly writing sessions to write their trauma narrative, after which a mental health professional read and responded to them by providing reflection, challenging cognitive distortions, and promoting cognitive flexibility. By August 2020, Mealer said, several hundred nurses had enrolled around the country, and some had requested the writing prompts to bring to their personal therapists. "It's sort of exposure therapy where they're having to confront those traumatic experiences that they've had to deal with in the work environment," she said. "But then there's also a cognitive processing component."

Katherine Virkstis, the managing director and senior research partner at the Advisory Board, said that storytelling is a key manner in which healthcare systems can boost engagement and help their staff find connection. She recalled the story of Ernest Shackleton, who was attempting to be the first to cross the Antarctic when his ship, Endurance, got stuck in an ice floe, and he had to lead his team out by foot. Despite drastically cutting back on supplies, Shackleton insisted that the ship's weatherman bring his banjo, as it brought the crew together. "That's something that some of the smart organizations are doing," said Virkstis, adding that it can be as simple as ninety-second storytelling at the beginning of a meeting, or more regular opportunities embedded into staff huddles and other workflow activities. "Building in that time for reflection and connection can be what makes the difference," she said.

8

Connecting Despite the Odds

Connection is the energy that is created between people when
they feel seen, heard, and valued.

—BRENÉ BROWN

Haider Warraich, a cardiologist in the Veterans Affairs (VA) system and
at Brigham and Women's Hospital in Boston, was struggling to find
common ground with a patient with bad heart failure, one who'd become
known as "difficult patient," when something changed. By observing a
nurse, who'd been spending much more time with the patient and had
developed a strong relationship with him, Warraich learned to take a different approach. "She knew what mattered to him most, what his wife's
name was, what his dog's name was, what he really wanted from his life,"
Warraich said. "It was really through her that I saw: What language do I
need to speak to this patient? What are the things that I need to emphasize when I talk to him? And just understanding better what he wanted
out of his interaction with the heath system and the medical team." Warraich made an effort to shift his speech and manner, and just by doing

that, he was able to better connect with the patient and establish a treatment plan acceptable to them both.

In recent decades, clinicians have faced growing hurdles to finding connection—with each other, with their patients, and within the healthcare system as a whole. Many challenges have developed as the US medical system has morphed into a corporate behemoth, with a tangle of insurance providers, administrators, and pharmaceutical and supply companies all vying to meet their goals and profit margins. Others stem from long histories of abuse and neglect that have targeted minorities, particularly the African-American and Native American communities. Meanwhile, as technological advances have enhanced healthcare's ability to support those suffering from serious brain injuries or organ failure, medical professionals have been tasked with finding unique ways to engage with patients on life support, in comas, or in disordered states of consciousness. During the COVID-19 pandemic, many clinicians were especially challenged with overcoming the distance created by personal protective equipment, oxygen masks, and isolation measures.

Physicians such as Warraich, whose time with patients has been increasingly limited by the evolving medical system, have learned to set boundaries, question systemic irregularities, and draw on nurses as a resource. While a 2020 Gallup poll found that the public's trust of both nurses and physicians had improved during the pandemic, nurses were rated the most honest and ethical of fifteen professions for the nineteenth year running. "A nurse's approach is just inherently so different from a physician's," Warraich said. "It leads to that stronger relationship rooted in trust and empathy."

Letting Patients Take the Lead

Jamie Lynn Leslie, an assistant professor at the University of Cincinnati College of Nursing in Ohio, spent eight or nine years as a home health nurse prior to taking on her academic role—mostly in Chicago, followed by two years in Cincinnati. During that time, she learned what strengthened or weakened trust with her patients, many of whom were recovering from orthopedic surgeries. She found that it was important to display transparency by documenting outcomes, and to "do what you say you're going to do, when you're going to do it." While Leslie couldn't promise to arrive at a specific time, patients were pleased with a two-hour window (a four-hour timeframe was too much)—often, she'd post their upcoming appointment on their refrigerator. Leslie learned the most from her mistakes—such as the nearly blind woman that she thought she'd helped by setting up her many medications in a pill container, with each day identified in braille. But when Leslie returned the following week, the patient had pulled the whole thing apart, and her pills were strewn across the table. "I kind of realized that she didn't trust me," Leslie said. "She was pretty upset, and I was upset." They reverted to the patient's original approach, which involved placing a colorful circle on top of each bottle that was bright enough for her to see. While this method didn't allow Leslie to confirm that the patient had been taking her medications correctly, she relied on blood pressure measurements and other vital signs. "I had to let her do it the way that she wanted, and I just had to trust her," Leslie said. "You really have to let patients take the lead."

Early on in her career, Leslie collaborated with two colleagues to analyze the literature on trust between patients and registered nurses—the resulting paper, published in *Home Healthcare Now* in 2016, found that antecedents to trust included meeting a need; respect; attention to time; continuity of care; and the effectiveness of the initial visit. Attributes of trust were identified as communication, connection, and reciprocity, while outcomes included improved collaboration and adaptation to illness; security; and additional trust.

To establish trust on an initial visit, Leslie found that it was important to invest time—her first appointments generally took at least an hour, while follow-up visits lasted roughly thirty minutes. "I really tried to just have a presence—to just be with them, and spend enough time so that I could see what they're doing," Leslie said. "Let them lead and ask a lot of questions." While this was typical to the home healthcare field, Leslie benefitted from the fact that she was working part-time, allowing her to limit home visits to six to eight a day, and to turn down new patients—a luxury not afforded full-time nurses, who often saw ten. "I couldn't imagine how you could do the same quality work if you were full-time," said Leslie, who spent three days a week visiting patients, while following up with phone calls to physicians, physical therapists, and social workers.

For most healthcare workers employed by hospitals or practice groups, spending sixty minutes with a patient is flat-out impossible. David Thom, a family medicine physician and clinical professor at Stanford Medicine who's published several papers on physician-patient trust, said "more time" is the number one institutional factor that would improve connection. "It's very difficult to have the kind of relationship that most of us want with patients if you're constrained to thirty-minute visits regardless of the situation, to having our schedules so packed that a patient can't get in to see us," he said. Thom, who finished his residency just as the US healthcare system was increasingly embracing managed care in the 1990s, found that in his experience, the change created concern that physicians would be driven more by profit than by patient care, while positioning primary care physicians as gatekeepers to resources such as specialists—causing some patients to approach him in an antagonistic manner. "That was a big shock," said Thom, whose neatly-trimmed white hair and goatee frame kindly features. Meanwhile, the availability of the Internet, combined with a growing distrust of the medical system, motivated many patients to come in armed with their own information—and sometimes, misinformation—to demand specific prescriptions or referrals without seeking Thom's input, while others were so passive he found it difficult to engage them in their own care. "A lot of what I do is just try to give patients more autonomy, more ability to direct the relationship and make more of an effort to define goals more clearly so that expectations are realistic and not unrealistic," Thom said.

One of the key hurdles to allowing providers enough time to establish trust with patients has been the growing cost of healthcare, and organizations' inability—or unwillingness—to prioritize the clinician-patient relationship. The US has been struggling with how to organize and pay for healthcare since the mid-twentieth century; this struggle has, in part, been exacerbated by the national decision to categorize healthcare as a market-based good. Following World War II, President Harry Truman proposed a national, taxpayer-funded healthcare system to cover all Americans. These efforts failed, due to opposition from Republicans and Southern Democrats in Congress, and from the American Medical Association (AMA), which spent millions of dollars to campaign against the initiative, labeling it "socialized medicine." As employer-based health coverage grew and private plans raised premiums, policymakers rallied to support the poor and elderly through the creation of Medicare and Medicaid in 1965. Healthcare costs continued to rise, prompting President Richard Nixon's administration to propose the Health Maintenance Organization Act of 1973, which invested millions in establishing and expanding HMOs, and required many employers to offer HMO coverage to encourage competition. This led to the rise of managed care, a series of techniques to control medical costs and provide health insurance while improving quality, that were initially employed by HMOs and later embraced by the healthcare system at large. Since then, the US healthcare system has operated under an increasingly corporatized model, influenced by the oft-competing interests of insurance providers, hospital administrators, corporate CEOs, and other players, and often making it more difficult for doctors to focus on what they identify as their desired priority: patient care.

Warraich said that he believes the fee-for-service payment model, which was traditionally in use with family care providers and has now been expanded into the long, complicated bills issued by healthcare organizations, has driven inappropriate practices, such as physicians failing to do due diligence when over-prescribing opioids, and is contributing to a breakdown in trust. "I think in medicine in general, we do need a deep cleanse—our field has been deeply corrupted by these pharmaceutical companies and device-makers," said Warraich, who aims to establish trust with his patients by ensuring he never accepts money from interests that could taint his decisions. (In an attempt to assist patients in determining which doctors or institutions are reliable, the federal government has even established an "Open Payments" searchable database to identify those who've accepted such funds.) Regardless, the fee-for-service model means that many institutions benefit from excess procedures. "The more services they provide people, whether they're beneficial or not, the more they get paid," Warraich said.

In recent years, there's been a push toward value-based care, in which reimbursement is based on the quality of care provided, measured by metrics such as patient satisfaction scores and positive outcomes. Yet this model has its own issues, including the fact that patient satisfaction can be driven by factors other than the quality of medical care—such as the inability to obtain pain medication, or administrative frustrations—while its adoption in tandem with the fee-for-service model can only create further billing complications. A national 2018 survey found that 43 percent of doctors believed value-based care would negatively impact the doctor-patient relationship, while 61 percent believed it would negatively impact their practice.

Adam Gaffney, a practicing pulmonary and critical care physician and public health researcher who teaches at Harvard Medical School, advocates for a single-payer healthcare system that he believes would better support both patients and physicians. To adopt such a system, he said, would eliminate many of the administrative tasks that absorb physicians' time. "You have a very large number of insurance plans, each with their own rules and regulations and exclusions," said Gaffney, who was formerly the president of the nonprofit Physicians for a National Health Program. "You have onerous prioritization procedures that again differ from insurance to insurance. You have a very complex billing system. So just all of that—put that together and it really does add to a huge amount of clerical burden." There are two ways to design a single-payer system, Gaffney said: To retain the current billing system and have healthcare organizations bill the government instead of the insurance companies; or preferably, to follow the course of Canada and Scotland and pay hospitals' whole budgets. "It allows them to slim down this whole [administrative] apparatus, which is 25 percent of hospital revenue, but it would also allow them to within their system operating budget actually increase provision of healthcare," Gaffney said. For physicians, this would mean they're salaried and do not have to worry about billing, prior authorizations, and other insurance-related negotiations, Gaffney said, adding: "I'm somewhat pessimistic about radically changing physicians' work under our current financing system."

While the HMO model hasn't resolved all paperwork challenges—and HMO physicians commonly complain that they are not allotted enough time for patient visits—it generally separated physician salaries from services provided, reduced the billing burden, and set quality standards. Rodney Hood, who was not initially a proponent of managed care, found that it improved quality because providers were forced to meet certain criteria on preventative measures such as pap smears, prostate cancer screenings, and colonoscopies. Hood, who previously owned an independent physicians association called MultiCultural IPA, said that because it was run by physicians rather than administrators, the doctors were focused on making needed changes to streamline patient services rather than simply saving money. "If it's done in a humane way, it works," he said.

Humanity on a corporate level must nevertheless filter down to a human level to have significant effect—including the formation of doctor-patient trust, particularly in underserved communities. As president of the Multicultural Health Foundation and CEO and managing partner at Care View Medical Group, Hood has been working to build trust in the Black community he serves. "When you break it down by ethnicity, Blacks continually have the lowest level of trust," he said, referencing not only Tuskegee, but repeated atrocities going back to Marion Sims's experimentation on African-American women during slavery. "Historically, they have been not only treated with disrespect, but inhumanely." As a result, Hood has struggled to get his Black patients to accept the COVID-19 vaccines developed by Pfizer and Moderna. Early on, Hood recognized that a vaccine was going to be critical to ending the pandemic, but he also realized that while African-Americans were being hit the hardest, they were the least likely to trust vaccination. At one point, Hood said, a patient asked him "about this vaccine, this Warp Speed, you know, with Trump. Are you going to take that?" Hood realized that he wasn't sure about it, either—he needed more information. Along with some colleagues at the National Medical Association (NMA), an organization of Black physicians, Hood proposed the formation of an NMA task force composed of Black specialists in vaccines and infectious disease to conduct an independent study and make recommendations. The task force approved the vaccines, and after studying the science, Hood, who became a strong believer, was vaccinated in January 2021.

As cofounder of the San Diego County COVID-19 Equity Task Force, Hood has also been instrumental in bringing more COVID-19 testing sites to underserved communities. Initially, it was hard for people in San Diego's low-income, diverse neighborhoods referred to as "south of eight" to get tested, so the task force worked with the county to open more test sites in highly impacted areas. At one site, the Tubman Chavez Community Center, people were initially required to make appointments, which they did—but less than 80 percent showed up. County officials consulted with Hood, concerned there wasn't enough need, but Hood convinced them to offer walk-in testing, after which the site became very busy. "It's an example of listening to folks who are in the community," Hood said. "These folks have got other issues going on their lives and are not always the best at keeping appointments because of those issues."

Hood, who is an advocate for including more Black participants in clinical trials—and who would have participated in COVID-19 vaccine trials himself had a recent flu shot not disqualified him—encouraged his patients to do so, and has worked to further vaccination efforts through the dissemination of videos featuring trusted messengers such as Black doctors and nurses. He acknowledged that the burden of bridging the gap between the two communities can take its toll. "There's a lot of chronic stress" on Black doctors, Hood said—and simply not enough of them to go around. While he advocates improving representation in medicine through targeted—and broadened—medical school recruitment efforts and pipeline creation, Hood emphasized that it's important for clinicians of other ethnicities to develop the ability to establish trust with Black patients. To do so, he said, they should simply show respect— by demonstrating care and empathy; by addressing their patients in a courteous manner; and by not talking down to them or becoming angry or upset if they decide not to follow recommendations. "I make it a point of sometimes spending more time asking the patient about their family, about what their likes are, and talking about issues that are not related to the medical visit," Hood said. "And I think all that leads to developing trust and respect."

Seeking Personhood

While healthcare workers can often face significant challenges in establishing effective communication with conscious patients, working with patients with traumatic brain injuries or disorders of consciousness poses uniquely trying circumstances. How does one determine if a patient is conscious? When a patient's brain shows some activity, might they be awake even if their body is immobile? What therapies are most helpful? Can they recover? Fortunately, there are scientists and clinicians who are actively seeking to answer these questions—often, with profoundly insightful results.

In the late 1990s, neuroscientist Adrian Owen was working on brain imaging techniques in the UK when a colleague asked him to see a patient named Kate, whose acute disseminated encephalomyelitis had left her in a vegetative state. They decided to show Kate images of her friends and families while she lay in a PET scanner and were shocked by what they found: her brain responded in the exact same manner as that of a normal, healthy person. "Everybody thought I was bonkers to bother putting a vegetative patient into a brain scanner," said Owen, who'd been hoping to get some insight into which areas of the brain were most damaged and why, but was "completely floored" by the results. "It just really got me going, to be honest. It completely changed my career."

Over the following decades, Owen continued to scan patients with traumatic brain injuries and disorders of consciousness—using PET scans, fMRI technology and more recently, a portable scanner called functional near-infrared spectroscopy (fNIRS). In his book, *Into the Gray Zone: A Neuroscientist Explores the Mysteries of the Brain and the Border between Life and Death*, Owen outlined his innovative approaches: he's placed patients in an fMRI scanner and then asked them to imagine specific scenarios such as playing tennis or walking through their house that were easily measured with imaging. When he had them imagine one scenario or the other as "yes" or "no" answers to questions, some were able to do so. Essentially, he had provided them with a way to communicate.

Yet this also created some ethical dilemmas. The scans were time and resource intensive, and only a limited number of questions could be asked. Which ones should they be? Whose interests should they serve—that of the patient, or of science, which was seeking to benefit many more such patients? Sometimes, Owen was able to make these interests overlap—such as when a patient's family members wanted to know whether the patient was aware of the birth of a niece and other recent family events. Owen shaped it into an exploration of how much memory was intact—and found the patient was able to recall everything, both before and after his injury. Thanks to Owen's research, and that of others, it's now widely accepted that one in five vegetative patients is likely conscious, while studies show that vegetative states may be misdiagnosed more than 40 percent of the time. More recently, Owen's efforts involve scanning patients with acute brain injuries in the ICU in an effort to improve prognosis.

Other scientists are developing ways to help those with traumatic brain injuries recover, including Theresa Bender Pape, a clinical neuroscientist with a dual appointment at Edward Hines, Jr. VA Hospital and Northwestern University Feinberg School of Medicine in Chicago. Bender Pape, who speaks in the explanatory manner of someone used to navigating diverse disciplines, became interested in patients with traumatic brain injuries after her sister fell into a coma and she saw how little was understood about treatment, as well as "the trauma that my own family went through, the need for advocacy." She worked as a speech-language pathologist at a rehabilitation institute, and after obtaining her PhD in public health, Bender Pape engaged in post-doctoral work and training in traumatic brain injury outcomes. Now, she serves as the founding director of the Hines VA-Northwestern Neuroplasticity in Neurorehabilitation Lab, where she has been leading an interdisciplinary team of clinicians and scientists to test the therapeutic value of transcranial magnetic stimulation on patients with traumatic brain injuries.

Bender Pape learned early on to keep some emotional distance from her patients and their families. "You have to be close enough to provide compassionate care," she said, "but I can't go in and help a family member process something emotionally, that's going too far in." Still, she is deeply touched by positive outcomes, such as a patient named Laura whose husband put together a video: Set to music, Laura is first pictured as a beautiful, animated mother; then, after being hit by a car while riding her bicycle, she's observed in bed in a minimally conscious state; and finally, she regains enough function to stand, speak, and even read. "The hair stands up on the back of your neck, and you remember why you're figuring out this really complicated problem," Bender Pape said.

Bender Pape does often establish long-term relationships with patients and their families, who continue to seek her input and advocacy over the years—and their insight has informed her approach. The mother of a patient she saw as a post-doctoral researcher—who, two decades later, still comes into her lab to support other family members—taught Bender Pape to look for personhood. "What they perceive as meaningful change is very different than what I perceive as meaningful change," Bender Pape said of family caregivers, who enabled her to recognize when someone's personality began emerging through minimal actions. One aspect of Bender Pape's current research explores what meaningful progress means to both clinicians and caregivers, and aims to create a behavioral hierarchy of recovery—often, these indicators involve the emergence of personhood. Bender Pape noticed Laura's personhood emerging one morning when she entered the room and greeted her. "She looks at me and goes—a fist bump, and then the rain dropping," Bender Pape laughed, raising her own fist in emulation before allowing her fingers to sprinkle downward. "That's personhood." Laura wasn't yet verbal, but her sense of humor also began to emerge. "I'm a bit of a sarcastic person, and she would smile at my jokes," Bender Pape said.

Due to the lack of theory and research, as well as the challenges posed by the patient population, Bender Pape described her field as "swimming in ambiguity." She stressed the importance of humility and respectful teamwork, and wants society to know how little attention and resources the population has received—despite the fact that there are nearly 3 million traumatic brain injuries in the US every year, and it could happen to anyone. In addition to her research, advocating for patients, mentoring, writing scientific publications and disseminating information, Bender Pape has even begun to talk to people on airplanes about her work— something she was motivated to do after an aspiring young neuroscientist expressed interest in the images on her computer—and has continued in an effort to connect her patients to society at large. She believes caregivers need financial support, while patients—most of whom are denied rehab by their insurance—need access to continuous care. "I guess I would like society to know about the forgotten people," she said.

Patients who are able to access rehab end up under the care of someone like Kenneth Ngo, the youthful medical director of Brooks Rehabilitation Hospital in Jacksonville, Florida, who heads their brain injury program and has spent a decade seeing four hundred to five hundred patients with brain injuries a year. Clinically, Ngo finds his patients interesting, while behaviorally they can be rather fun. "When a patient has a severe brain injury they can be very inappropriate," said Ngo, laughing as he recalled a patient who'd recently complimented him on his looks—along with every other male staff on the floor—and later tried to grab a male therapist's butt. "Every day is different, and every patient's responses and behavior are different." With the inappropriate patient, Ngo developed a plan to help curb the behaviors "because in her mind, she doesn't know that those are inappropriate." She was injured less than a month prior, and was likely to recover, he said.

While most of Ngo's patients have suffered traumatic brain injuries from causes such as falls, accidents, gunshots, or abuse, some have also suffered nontraumatic brain injuries, which could be caused by a brain tumor, or loss of oxygen due to a heart attack. Over the years, Ngo has learned not to delve too deeply into the cause of their injury—unless it's something he needs to know for discharge purposes, such as spousal abuse. He'd rather not know if a patient had been driving under the influence of drugs or alcohol, or was otherwise at fault. "Do I blame him?" Ngo asked. "Well, I'm not going to treat him any differently. His sweet mom is still there." Often, Ngo connects quite significantly with the families and will regularly text them to keep in touch or ask questions on behalf of patients who can't communicate.

Ngo typically tries to figure out what patients were like before their injuries, which allows him to better connect with patients while also recognizing personhood when it emerges. "Was he a goofball? Was he the life of the party? Did he like football?" Ngo said. "That makes it more personal, that it's a person that we're treating, and not treating the condition." Part of the rehab involves figuring out what the patient can do now; it may not be returning to a prior career such as engineering. Sometimes, patients can find a different vocation; others can volunteer; still others may be unable to work but still have the ability to laugh and connect with loved ones. When a patient doesn't make an expected level of recovery, Ngo sees it more as a problem to solve than as a failure, while dramatically positive outcomes can be invigorating. Still, certain patients can cause some distress, such as the thirty-one-year-old man whose car was hit by an eighteen-wheeler from behind, leaving him in a vegetative state several months later. He had two children who were the same age as Ngo's children; they even had similar names. "His life will never be the same again—he will not be the Dad that his kids know," Ngo said. "I thought of him often, just because it kind of hit close to home."

Jennifer Quartano, a clinical specialist in neurologic physical therapy who teaches at the Brooks Rehabilitation Institute of Higher Learning, was inspired to pursue physical therapy after injuring her knee as a teenager and managing to recover without surgery. She's worked in acute care, the ICU, and in outpatient settings, which has given her the opportunity to view patients all along the continuum of care. Sometimes, Quartano has found herself challenged by patients whose families hoped for impossible outcomes, such as a seven-year-old girl who'd been injured in a car accident when the father was driving. Quartano walked into the room to find the little girl unconscious and buried in tubes—half of her long, brown hair had been shaved for emergency surgery, and her face, swollen and bruised, was fading to a deep yellow. When Quartano asked the father about his goals for his daughter, he said he wanted her to finish school, get married, and have a good job. "It kind of just hit me," Quartano said. "I was thinking: sit up, walk—those are the kinds of things we usually hear." By the time the girl left the facility, she was still pretty low functioning, but Quartano had been able to help the father see what she could do—squeeze a hand, hold her head up on her own, or lean against someone for support; times when her personhood would reveal itself. "Even though that affection was different than it was before, she was still able to show little pieces of that, and little pieces of her own personality coming through," Quartano said.

Quartano considers a physical therapist's role with vegetative or minimally conscious patients to be partly to provide treatment, such as physical movement, but also to look for a response from the individual and to help the family understand what it means—to differentiate between purposeful and reflexive movement. "Oftentimes we get involved in things like rolling over in bed, or rolling a ball, or little things that might not seem much like therapy but are very much therapy," Quartano said. "Brushing their hair, getting all those knots out of it, seeing even if they'll grimace when I pull on their hair accidentally." Quartano always makes sure to speak directly to the patient, rather than about them, and uses short, simple commands when seeking a response. She often thinks of *The Diving Bell and the Butterfly*, a book written by Jean-Dominique Bauby, the former editor-in-chief of French *Elle*, who experienced locked-in syndrome following a stroke; he was fully conscious, and communicated the words for his book by blinking his left eye. "That's one of the things that influences me as I think about how I communicate and what I communicate," Quartano said.

When she has a patient with heart-wrenching circumstances, such as the seven-year-old girl, Quartano leans on her team, who understands what she's going through, and sets aside time to exercise or otherwise disengage. "Emotionally it can be very, very challenging," she said. She takes comfort from the success stories that come back for follow-up—but realizes that many patients go home to live a very different life. "It's a balance of making sure we don't get overly attached because there's always another patient that needs our help," Quartano said. "If I give all of myself to this family and this situation then I have nothing left for the next one that comes in the door."

"It Was So Therapeutic"

Doctors, nurses, therapists, and others working in critical care often rely heavily on patients' family members to connect with the patients themselves. These third-party relationships enable clinicians to navigate the challenges posed by disorders of consciousness, incommunicative states, and ventilators—and can become quite intimate. During the COVID-19 pandemic, some clinicians went above and beyond to keep family members engaged, finding unique ways to sidestep the barriers created by PPE and social distancing. This level of engagement can mean that the loss of a patient, or an otherwise undesirable outcome, hits even closer to home. But while some practitioners advocate keeping a certain emotional distance, others have found that joining family members in the grieving process provides an outlet and enlivened sense of meaning.

DaiWai Olson, a neurological critical care nurse and professor in the neurology department at the University of Texas Southwestern Medical Center, has focused his research around understanding how nursing care contributes to outcomes for patients with acquired brain injuries. Olson began working in a general ICU in the 1980s, and since they began specializing in the 1990s, has spent the past twenty-five years focusing on neurological critical care. "Caring for an unconscious patient is a very intimate act," Olson said, adding that he often reflects on what he would want if roles were reversed—such as being repositioned in bed, being bathed, or having his teeth brushed and hair combed—in addition to the regular nursing duties such as checking blood pressure, brain pressure, and handling feeding and toileting needs. Often, he said, nurses will stand and scan the unconscious patient's room to identify what's required. "When I walk by and see one of my fellow nurses standing in a room, I know how hard they're working," Olson said. "It's actually a purposeful, intent-driven process."

Olson spends a lot of time talking to families—not just immediate relations, but also patients' connected circle of friends—to find out what they liked. Did they like lying on their left side? What kind of music did they listen to? Did they enjoy sunlight, or prefer dimmer rooms? Did they like to talk about Hollywood gossip, or football? "These are cues and clues, and nurses look for these and then we incorporate them," Olson said. The mother of one young man, a gang member who'd been shot in the head, was certain that he'd want to listen to her pastor's recorded speeches 24/7, but the patient's friends and fellow gang members advised otherwise. They described him as rather introverted, and as someone who didn't often listen to music, so Olson and the patient's care team would turn the TV on and off and would talk to each other rather than to the patient directly to make him feel more comfortable. When his mother visited, they'd put on the pastor's recording. "He did do fairly, surprisingly well," Olson said. "But when he did start to come out and emerge from his consciousness disorder, he didn't reach for the cassette tape that mom had left him." Other patients who've spent years in minimally conscious states have complained after recovering that what had once been their favorite music became tedious; one told her mother that she never wanted to hear Celine Dion, formerly her favorite musician, again.

Olson—who is a member of the Curing Coma Campaign, which seeks to develop and implement coma treatment strategies—imagines patients in a coma as being behind a wall. "You've got to figure out the loose bricks to help them get through that wall to a conscious state," he said. (Often, family members play a critical part of this process; Bender Pape's earlier research found that hearing stories from familiar voices, such as family members, led to gains in attention and awareness.) Once, Owen noticed a patient named Toby, who'd fallen into a coma due to a brain infection, had been rubbing his thumb and forefinger together repeatedly, to the point that it was causing damage. Olson took the remote control for the television and used it to separate the two appendages. The next day, he moved it around. "We play with our patients," Owen said. "We don't mean it derogatorily, but like you do with a one-year-old whose brain is emerging." Soon, Toby was turning the television on and off; a couple of weeks later he was changing channels. Then, one day, he started looking toward the TV. "That was his loose brick in the wall," Owen said. "This is the thing that worked for him."

Olson said that he's always emotionally impacted by the work that he does, and that he's okay with that. Often, he sees minimally conscious, vegetative, or coma patients move into long-term acute care facilities or return home with a family caregiver. Sometimes, they surprise him—like the patient in a vegetative state whose husband adamantly refused to remove life support, and who eventually recovered enough to ride a horse and speak. Other times, he's had to explain to families that their loved one is rotting from the inside before they decide to stop treatment. "It's not my job to tell you when to give up or when to stop," said Olson, who takes comfort from being there for patients in any way he can, as well as appreciating well-intentioned humor when it emerges. "It's my job to make sure that you have all the knowledge possible to make your decision on an individual basis."

While connections to patients in minimally conscious states and their families can be heartwarming, they can also present a challenge when that patient doesn't recover. Dustin Money, a specialist in extracorporeal membrane oxygenation (ECMO) at the University of Virginia Health System, worked as a respiratory therapist for seven years before going into ECMO—a relatively new technology that essentially operates the patient's heart and lungs, pumping their blood outside the body to oxygenate it. Money, who also works part-time as a researcher, spends three twelve-to-sixteen-hour shifts a week in the pediatric, neonatal, or adult cardiovascular ICU and has taken on much more responsibility: he's not only managing the technology, but also coordinating other aspects of patient care. It's also much more intimate, because Money has just one or two patients at a time, often for extended periods—and, not uncommonly, they're children.

Money often finds himself become more attached to these patients—such as the four-year-old girl who was accidently run over by her aunt and then developed a COVID-19 infection. "You get in these situations sometimes where you just get really invested," said Money, a heavyset man with a teddy bear-like quality who has two children of his own. Money worked overtime to care for the girl, who was sedated and paralyzed on ECMO—a month later, she was finally making progress. Money made sure she was bathed and braided her hair. Early on in his ECMO years, he'd become very attached to another girl, a six-year-old with flu pneumonia, who'd died. "When you have a tiny little girl that kind of looks like your daughter, you just want to be like her Dad and take care of her," said Money, who'd brought in his daughter's pink nail polish to paint her nails. "It's a lot harder emotionally, being in my current role."

Some ECMO patients are receiving cardiac and respiratory support while their heart or lungs heal, while others are waiting for an organ transplant, heart implant, or other therapy; what Money tries to avoid is "building a bridge to nowhere." When a patient continues to decline, or multiple organ systems begin to fail, the time can come to withdraw support. And while doctors are typically tasked with these conversations, Money often finds himself translating for the family, or even preparing them in advance. "Since you know the family and the patient so intimately, the families themselves look to you for answers," he said. "I enjoy trying to keep family members and patients on the same page and letting them know ahead of time what's coming." Still, Money acknowledges that the job can be incredibly stressful, particularly when he has to withdraw life support for someone whose family he's come to know well or when he's been involved in traumatic situations, such attempting to put a young pregnant woman on ECMO during an attempted resuscitation and emergency C-section—both of which failed. "I've gone through the gamut of maybe drinking too much," he said. "I've gone through the gamut of maybe withdrawing from my own family for a few days so I can process it. Sometimes it haunts you for a little while."

Christopher Cox, a critical care doctor and associate professor of medicine at Duke University, said he enjoys the opportunity to work with families as well as their patients as medical director of the ICU. Often, when the decision is made to intubate a patient, Cox said, the patient is too ill to speak, so much of the discussion occurs with family members.

A ninety-year-old with COVID-19 pneumonia who's rapidly worsening may not find the treatment worthwhile, while other situations are less clear-cut. Cox found that the pandemic really highlighted the need for people to have goals-of-care conversations early on, so that the family would know what they'd want. "It's much better than when you're gasping for breath in extremis, and some person you've never met before is saying, 'Hey, do you want to be on this life support machine or not?'" he said. "More often than not, that's kind of how it goes down." Cox has found himself in the odd position of navigating end-of-life discussions with people on their first visit. "You have to do what's almost like rapid speed-dating to kind of get to know each other and figure out what's important to them," he said.

Sometimes patients on life support are sedated, or even chemically paralyzed, while others remain awake or partially conscious. "It makes it easier to get them off the machine when they're awake, so that's the aim," Cox said. He estimates that typically at least half, and sometimes three-quarters, of the patients in his ICU are on life support such as ventilators; in his experience, about 75 percent survive. The sickest are often in the ICU for weeks, and Cox makes an effort to play music that they like or provide a comforting voice—particularly during the COVID-19 pandemic, when loved ones were often unable to visit. His team would Facetime with families, and Cox called the families and updated them while examining a patient or asked them if there was a message that he could relay. "We really try to get creative with those sorts of things," he said. "We think it's important."

Joey Traywick, a nurse in Billings, Montana, also employed creative means to connect with his patients and their families despite the barriers posed by COVID-19. Traywick was nearing retirement in February 2020 when he took a seemingly low-key spot on a new floor at his hospital, an observation unit for patients with chest pain—a month later, the unit had become the hospital's dedicated, isolated COVID-19 unit. By fall, their caseload had grown exponentially, and patients were much more critically ill. Traywick was decked out in full PPE—a gown, mask, face shield, and gloves, in addition to his glasses—and had to find ways to reach his patients, who were wearing BiPAP oxygen masks and trying to speak over the loud, sucking sound of a negative pressure HEPA air filter. Often, Traywick would bring family Christmas cards in to show his patients: "This is me," he'd say, pointing at his open-mouthed smile, red baseball cap, and jean jacket, with his arms around his wife and three children. Often, he'd use a dry erase board to ask patients if he could order them breakfast, or how they'd slept. He'd also ask to see photos of them and their families. "Nine out of ten have them right there" on their cell phones, he said.

Traywick found himself deeply drawn into family discussions and dynamics—family members informed him of whom the patient would want to talk to, and which calls to avoid. Many patients couldn't figure out how to use the hospital iPads, and so Traywick would assist by meeting the family in the lobby with the iPad, and using it to call a cell phone in the room. Traywick would find himself repeating messages that a patient couldn't hear: "She said, 'I love you.'" Once, he found himself holding the iPad for two small children while their young, dying mother cried. Sometimes, family members would pray for their loved one over the iPad, or ask for or offer forgiveness—with Traywick right there, in the middle. "Incredibly intimate, sacred, holy places that you shouldn't really be there for," he said. Other times, Traywick had to decide what not to relay, such as when a terrified patient, who was struggling to breathe, was trying to rip off their mask—a not uncommon situation for those who had decided against intubation and remained on his unit rather than going to the ICU. "The traumatic part of it is the balance between what you tell the family and what you don't," he said.

Many of Traywick's patients were Native American—mostly, Northern Cheyenne—and their extended families, some forty or fifty people, would often congregate in a circle in the parking lot or nearby park, holding vigil. When a patient Traywick had become close to, J. D. Old Mouse—the traditional flute maker for the Northern Cheyenne people—died in the ICU, his family called Traywick in the hospital, and he went down to the parking lot to see them. He thought they might be angry, or frustrated. Instead, they put Traywick in the middle of the circle and prayed for him.

"It was just devastating," he said. "I was just on my knees, sobbing. Not only because he had passed, but because they were so gracious." After the family left to accompany the hearse to the funeral home, Traywick went home and held his own ritual—a fire in the backyard—as his wife and children watched from the house (Traywick often lived in the basement during the pandemic to prevent contagion). Later, Old Mouse's wife Amy invited Traywick to breakfast with her son and gave him a beaded lanyard—graded shades of fiery colors, interspersed with black, white, and blue—in thanks. "She said, 'Look, I took a beading class because I wanted to learn to bead so I could make this for you,'" said Traywick, who was incredibly touched. "It was so therapeutic."

Traywick's deep connections to patients and families have also allowed him to grieve in real time—and, he believes, have protected him against burnout. While the majority of Traywick's patients recovered, by February 2021, he had personally counted twenty-seven who'd died from the disease—sometimes, in his unit; sometimes, like Old Mouse, in the ICU. "I'm the last one that got to be with them, most of the time," Traywick said. He often sat with the young mother to watch her favorite show, *Grey's Anatomy*; when the doctor said there was nothing more they could do, he stayed after his shift to do so. "She's crying and I'm crying," Traywick said. "We connected on the level of *Grey's Anatomy*—watching people die on TV, and her realizing: that's going to be me." As Traywick also holds a degree in theater, he'd often ask dying patients if they had a favorite song. One patient requested "You Are My Sunshine"; another, "Amazing Grace." For an Elvis fan, he sang "Love Me Tender."

Traywick has listed the name of each patient who's died on a yellow legal pad and has kept every card, every note, every gift. "We try to do that little bit on our floor, when someone's passing, to connect them with family, but it's a miserable, pathetic substitute for actually being there," he said. "They deserve to be commemorated." Sometimes, though, Traywick wonders if he's overreacting—such as keeping the nail clippers he last used on Old Mouse to himself. Or when he lost a simple, black bracelet that a family member had made for him when jogging, and he obsessively reran the same six-mile route for days afterward, searching for it.

"At some point I would imagine this intensity will have to wane," said Traywick, who can relate to the Vietnam veterans in *The Body Keeps the Score: Brain, Mind, and the Body in the Healing of Trauma*, a book by Bessel van der Kolk that explores how trauma reshapes both the body and the brain. The veterans recalled the war as some of the most intense times of their lives—and yet also the most meaningful in terms of connections to their fellow soldiers. Traywick was struck by one veteran named Tom who didn't want to lose his nightmares because, despite the terror, these dreams preserved his comrades' memories. Still, Traywick acknowledged that his method of memorializing is likely healthier. "I don't have nightmares, and I've got a lot of coworkers who do," Traywick said. "I think because I've connected to the families."

Getting to know patients' families provides many clinicians with both essential information and an opportunity to establish deep and meaningful relationships—building greater trust between healthcare workers and those they serve. These connections are often even more essential as patients approach the end of life and difficult decisions must be made. When should patients be put on ventilators or other forms of life support? At what point should life support be removed? What treatments are worth engaging in, and which will simply extend suffering? Fortunately, the emergence of palliative care, hospice, advance directives, and other end-of-life initiatives have made notable strides toward addressing these concerns. When utilized effectively, they can significantly reduce suffering for patients, as well as moral distress, empathy fatigue, and burnout for clinicians.

Part III

Changes in
End-of-Life Care

Confronting Death in Hospice

Death exists, not as the opposite but as a part of life.

—HARUKI MURAKAMI

Kevin Dieter has been a hospice doctor for more than thirty years. Still, Dieter's first introduction to hospice care, back in the late 1980s, was unexpected. He was just out of residency and running a small family medicine practice in Ohio when a ninety-three-year-old woman came in with multiple chronic conditions including heart failure, lung disease, hypothyroidism, diabetes, and arthritis. She was on a range of medications that were keeping her alive and wanted to stop taking them so that she could die naturally and no longer be a burden to her niece. "She said, 'I'm not depressed. I'm not trying to kill myself. I just don't want to keep taking these pills at this point in my life,'" said Dieter, whose dark eyebrows furrow in a thoughtful manner. "I started to panic a little bit. I'm thinking, 'I'm not really prepared for this.'"

Dieter screened the patient, whom he's since assigned the pseudonym "Ruth," for depression and other concerns, but she was insistent that she was going to do it on her own if he didn't help her. Dieter had

Ruth admitted to the hospital so that staff could address symptoms such as shortness of breath, irregular heartbeats, and peripheral edema as she went off her medications. "Over the next thirteen days, she became my most profound teacher," Dieter said. "First of all, she made me learn how to use medications like morphine and Ativan to keep her physically comfortable. But more importantly, she taught me about grace and dignity at the end of life. She taught me that each time I went into the room, I could not have my own agenda because really what played out was mostly not science. And it wasn't anything that I had a lot of control over." Ruth engaged in a life review—a common activity in which individuals look back on their lives to find meaning and resolution. She told Dieter indirectly what she'd appreciated about her healthcare providers in the past; said goodbye lovingly to her niece; and experienced visions of her deceased husband—something Dieter has since come to expect with patients approaching death, who commonly report seeing dead friends or relatives. "She actually showed me the way that people die naturally" without CPR or other last-resort treatments, Dieter said. A year or two later, the hospital where Dieter had admitted Ruth started its own hospice program and asked Dieter to be its medical director.

The concept of hospice care began to take hold in the United States in the mid-1970s, championed by the likes of Elisabeth Kübler-Ross, author of *On Death and Dying*, and Florence Wald, a nurse who founded the first US hospice in Connecticut based on Dame Cicely Saunders's model in the United Kingdom. Hospices, envisioned to provide holistic, coordinated, comprehensive, and compassionate care to the terminally ill, were independently formed until the mid-1980s, when Medicare began paying for hospice benefits. Fifteen years after the first hospice opened its doors, more than 1,000 hospice organizations existed nationwide; by 2018, there were more than 4,500. Hospice became an official medical subspecialty, providing physicians—including Dieter—the opportunity to become certified in hospice and palliative medicine. Now, patients who don't want to die amid the tubes and machinery typical of the ICU can focus on comfort measures while surrounded by family, friends, and caregivers, whether in an institution or at home. "I am a much better version of myself for having done hospice," Dieter said. "Sometimes it's very sad, but we actually get so much more out of doing this work than we give."

Hospice care enables clinicians to be present with patients as they die, rather than simply going through the motions of trying to save their lives. While this can be a powerful, uplifting, and even transformative experience for both patients and providers, it isn't always easy—or pretty. Some patients undergo extreme physical suffering that can't be fully alleviated, while others experience acute psychological or spiritual anguish. Clinicians working in hospice environments must navigate unique challenges—such as caring for the body and walking family members through the death and bereavement process. Simultaneously, they must develop effective ways to process their own experiences of ongoing grief and loss.

"An Unmet Need"

Americans can now receive hospice services at dedicated inpatient facilities, in hospitals, in nursing facilities, or at home. Hospice clinicians in hospitals must deal with the sudden onset of symptoms; those in home health may establish intimate connections with patients and their relatives; while nursing home staff often come to view residents, whom they can work with for years, as extended family. Each care setting brings its own unique stressors and challenges—ones that will only be exacerbated as Baby Boomers age. The population of Americans age sixty-five and older has been increasing by 10,000 a day, with all 73 million Baby Boomers expected to cross this threshold by 2030. Meanwhile, life expectancy at this stage has risen to over 19 years, up more than 7 years from 11.9 in the previous century. A focus group study of hospice workers suggested that administrators seeking to reduce burnout in the field should encourage self-care, provide appropriate coverage to allow clinicians time off, and address structural issues pertinent to administrative and communication concerns.

The majority of hospice patients die at home—the option most Americans state as their preference. While hospice care—which focuses on comfort measures and improving quality of life—can be highly beneficial for patients who are still undergoing treatment, Medicare only covers it for those who have waived treatment and have a diagnosis of six months or less to live. As a result, most patients receiving hospice care are dying. Of the 1.1 million Medicare beneficiaries who died in hospice during 2018, more than half were at home, 17.4 percent in nursing facilities, 12.3 percent in assisted living facilities, and 12.8 percent in hospice inpatient facilities. In terms of days that involved hospice care, more than half was provided within the home.

Lori Bishop, the vice president of palliative and advanced care at the National Hospice and Palliative Care Organization (NHPCO), said that many patients enter hospice fairly late in their illness; over half of patients receiving hospice care do so for less than a month. "That's a shame given the wealth of things that that benefit includes, that people are entitled to," Bishop said. "We have to start seeing hospice as a treatment option, instead of there's nothing left to do." Bishop, a former hospice nurse, said that one significant challenge faced by hospice providers in recent years is that the government's fiscal intermediaries have been scrutinizing more costly levels of care, meaning that patients at the end of life with acute symptoms may be transferred to a hospital or hospice facility and then forced to return home to a lower level of care once that symptom has been addressed—despite the fact that at that point they may not want to, as they could have only days, or even hours, to live. "It's awful," Bishop said, adding that clinicians were once able to recommend levels of care based on what was best for the patient—a norm she would like to see reinstated. "You hate to be the one to have those conversations" with family members, she said.

Jessamyn Tabakin, a general inpatient hospice social worker in a large hospital system in northern New Jersey, said that patients often come in seeking management for serious symptoms such as intractable pain, vomiting, dyspnea, bleeding, or other things that need intervention. While Tabakin doesn't develop extended relationships with patients over time, she often finds herself navigating a variety of family crises. "I've had experiences where there's been major estrangement and somebody's decided at the last second that they need to call in a family member, or there's some sort of revelation that happens at the bedside," she said. "Everyone is just kind of cracked open emotionally, which invites for a lot of incredible opportunities for growth—and also opportunity, in some cases, for extremely expressive emotion. . . . We have everything: screaming, yelling, throwing things, people on the floor." As a social worker, Tabakin finds herself creating space for patients and family members to express these strong emotions, while also providing support to other staff. "Many times that's just being an ear, or really asking someone when you're noticing that they're burnt out or there's some compassion fatigue," she said. "Sort of taking a minute and checking in."

Hospice care is typically provided by a multidisciplinary team including doctors, nurses, chaplains, social workers, counselors, home health aides, and trained volunteers—and while many report that they become accustomed to death and find it meaningful to participate in the process, all are impacted by the work that they do. In addition to managing patients' physical symptoms, the team provides emotional and spiritual support, medications, caregiver coaching, counseling, and bereavement care to patients and their families. In a small study published in *OMEGA – Journal of Death and Dying* in 2018, researcher Angela Ghesquiere found that home health aides at one urban New York hospice experienced a variety of emotional reactions to patient deaths, including sadness, shock, numbness, grief, and relief. Ways they found to cope included accepting the inevitability of death; making meaning by considering patients' deaths in light of spiritual beliefs or the fact that they were no longer suffering; and informal social support, particularly from other home health aides.

Home health aides are somewhat unique in that they spend extensive amount of time with their patients while making relatively low incomes that add additional stress. "They would really build these relationships," Ghesquiere said. "I think there was this real feeling of loss in a lot of cases, almost as if someone that they were close to on a personal level in their day-to-day life had passed away. And a lot of them, when we talked about it, would get kind of tearful and you could still see that the grief was still there, even if it had occurred a while ago." Many had little time to mourn—sometimes only hours, more often days—before they were assigned a new patient. And as they were out in the field, they weren't often able to participate in the hospice's weekday events to commemorate patient deaths or to connect with other staff members. They told Ghesquiere that they would benefit from a regular grief support group; training in interacting with bereaved family members; more sensitive communication around patient deaths; and education on self-care. A self-care day, organized by the hospice on a workday as part of the study, proved highly popular: it included chair massages; adult coloring exercises while listening to music; a self-care assessment and self-care tips; and a ritual in which the home health aides chose a stone or shell from a bowl that reminded them of a patient who'd died, shared something about the patient, and then placed it in another bowl. "They all spoke about how much that had been really helpful to them, to just have that space," Ghesquiere said.

Toni Miles, a professor of epidemiology and biostatistics at the University of Georgia College of Public Health who has created bereavement care guides for staff at nursing home and assisted living facilities, said that death in long-term care is often hidden or dismissed. When Miles first began researching how Georgia nursing home administrators handled deaths in 2015, she found that about half of them preferred to deal with it discreetly so as not to upset other residents, while the other half wanted to offer residents and staff the opportunity to say goodbye. "Some leadership will tell staffers, 'Oh, you know, it happens all the time so get used to it,'" Miles said. "You don't really want that because those people don't care. That's the path to burnout." Miles began training long-term care staff—as well as residents and families—on bereavement in late 2019, based on booklets, PowerPoint slides, and videos she'd developed. Once the COVID-19 pandemic hit, she transitioned to online webinars, as well as a toolkit mailed to all the nursing homes in Georgia. "This is an unmet need," Miles said of staff bereavement care. "People die that they care about. Some of them remind them of their relatives. So they need this." While many nursing homes lack memorial services, which can provide staff with an outlet in addition to residents and families, Miles said that one facility holds a service every Monday after Mother's Day. "People come together," she said. "They reminisce about everyone who died that year, you know, they light candles. Sometimes they release butterflies. And they honor the people who took care of them by washing their hands in essential oils." Miles added that some clinicians cry as their hands—the very hands that once bathed and cared for the patient—are washed. "When you deny that it happened, the staff member has no mechanism for releasing those emotions," she said.

Rowena Sheppard, a certified nursing assistant (CNA) at a nursing home and skilled rehab facility in Tennessee, said that she was inspired to become a CNA in 2016 after her father and her father-in-law died two days apart. While she'd cared for her father-in-law at the end of his life, Sheppard wasn't aware that her own father, back in the Philippines, was also dying. "I was devastated that I could not take care of my dad," she said. "And I just decided that maybe I should take care of other people."

Sheppard said she has worked both day and night shifts, during which she becomes close to residents as she assists them through activities such as eating and getting into and out of bed. Many of them have been there for the entire five years she's worked at the facility, and she views them "like extended family." They tell Sheppard that they love her, give her handmade cards or drawings—she has a collection of them now—and tell her that they've missed her. Even during the COVID-19 pandemic, Sheppard would touch and hug the residents. "They would always ask me," she said. "And I cannot say no. If you can say no to that, I think you're in the wrong profession." When Sheppard got home, she would take off all her clothes, put them in the washing machine, and take a shower to protect her husband and teenaged daughter.

Sheppard, who's experienced more patient deaths than she can count, has struggled with each one—especially early on in her career. "It's heartbreaking," she said. "Every time that happens I lose a part of myself. But I need to stay calm, because there are still other people who need me." Sheppard said that after a patient dies, she'll take a moment, consoling herself that they're in a better place, "laughing, talking, walking, dancing, even running—anything they want, because most of them could not even do that when they were still here." And when Sheppard engages in postmortem care, during which she cleans and prepares the body for viewing, she sees it as a final goodbye: an opportunity to present them, one last time, for their loved ones. She finds comfort in talking to her fellow CNAs and with her husband and daughter at home. And she takes heart when the facility offers small tokens of recognition—such as a cup with her name on it; T-shirts with the facility's logo; or free food for CNA week. "Without that being appreciated—what you do, and being acknowledged that you've done a good job and stuff like that—we're probably not going to make it," she said.

Not Turning Away

Since his experience with Ruth, Dieter, who is now the associate medical director of Hospice of the Western Reserve and works at the bedside of their forty-bed unit on the shores of Lake Erie in Cleveland, has become comfortable in walking people through the dying process, which can take anywhere from hours to months. He said that while there's a lot of variation, people who are dying typically become weaker and less functional—unable to get up and move around. "They naturally become unable to eat or drink," he said. "They may have significant physical pain depending upon the underlying illnesses that they have. They may get short of breath. They may have some anxiety, nausea, those kinds of things." Once patients begin what is called "active dying," they can emit a death rattle—a gurgling in the throat; their extremities can become discolored; or they can experience terminal restlessness and agitation. "Some people, truly, they lay down in their bed to die, and they do it, and they're comfortable," Dieter said. "And other people struggle and struggle and struggle, physically and emotionally and existentially, until the end."

Dieter has found that spiritual suffering can play as significant a role as physical suffering in people's discomfort. "We say that forgiveness is the common cold of spiritual pain and suffering at the end," Dieter said. "So when people need to forgive themselves for mistakes they've made and they can't do it, or they need to forgive others, or others need to forgive them. Or the toughest one is where they need to forgive God."

Some devout churchgoers become angry at God because they've developed cancer, he said. Other individuals struggle with a sense of hopelessness. Dieter has learned to make amends in his own life and to focus on forgiving others and himself. "If we address the things that may be important to us when we're dying and we take care of it when we're living and still healthy, not only does that make our dying process a lot easier, but it actually makes our life better," he said.

Spiritual care providers such as Pastor Jeffrey Thomas, a chaplain at HopeHealth in Rhode Island, assist patients to address some of these issues, while also reassuring families through some of the more concerning physical symptoms. Once, Thomas sat with a woman at the bedside of her husband, to whom she'd been married for more than seventy years, who was suffering from apnea. When he stopped breathing for prolonged periods, his wife became anxious, and wanted to call the hospital's nurse; Thomas reassured her that he was still breathing. "I was happy to have been able to be in the room with her," Thomas said. "No one else was there." The woman's husband eventually died, and years later she ran into Thomas leaving a retail store and enveloped him in a big hug before he could even see who she was. Often, Thomas will lead funeral services for those he's served; once, he performed a wedding for a man and his dying girlfriend. Yet Thomas rarely has time to process such events. "You finish that memorial service, and then you go do your next visit," he said. "There's no time for decompression or just kind of taking a moment to take a walk in the park."

Once a patient has been declared dead, hospice nurses, CNAs, and other professionals typically step in to provide postmortem care. Mikel Hand, an associate professor of nursing at the University of Southern Indiana, said that in addition to physical care of the deceased, postmortem care can involve psychosocial care and support for family and loved ones; administrative tasks such as paperwork and notifications; and ensuring that the body is properly identified. Healthcare staff—sometimes accompanied by a family member—will cleanse and reposition the body, removing intravenous catheters and other lines when appropriate while taking measures to prevent leakage of blood or other bodily fluids.

"I did find it affecting me, particularly in situations where I had long-term relationships with patients," said Hand, who during his more than thirty-year career performed postmortem care as a nurse in home care, hospice facility, and long-term care settings. "I felt sad. It certainly did have some effect on my sleep for a period of time. I guess in some ways I felt a little bit angry and frustrated. At the same time being realistic about the situation—what would the individual's quality of life have been if they were experiencing these complications and they were to live?"

Elisabeth Almerini, a hospice nurse who has provided postmortem care for some thirty years, mostly in New Jersey, often responds to calls from families when a patient has died in the home. She'll ascertain that the patient is dead and comfort the family, after which they'll usually leave the room. "For me, that's a very special, almost sacred time," said Almerini, who never rushes the postmortem care, but takes time to appreciate the process. "In a way, yours are the last hands to touch them before they go on the next part of their journey." Almerini said it can nevertheless be discomfiting to care for an individual with disfiguring wounds or tumors, such as the woman around her age with breast cancer who had lesions all over the front of her body. And the first time she had to provide postmortem care, early on in her career at an urban New York hospital, Almerini had to do it alone, and worried that she might be hurting the patient, or even that the patient could wake up. "Things will kind of flop in a way that you don't want them to," said Almerini, who struggled to lift the patient's body and encase it in the shroud, and was concerned by mishaps in transporting the body to a stretcher. Still, Almerini's greatest challenge in hospice care has not been dealing with death, but rather the increasingly heavy documentation burden required to meet stringent Medicare requirements. For every half-hour with a patient, Almerini has to spend double that time documenting the visit—a factor that contributed to her decision to stop working for a couple of years, and more recently, to reduce her hours to less than twenty per week.

MaryEllen Kirkpatrick, the former residence chef at the Zen Hospice Project's Guest House in San Francisco (which closed in 2018), started as a volunteer and ended up staying four years. "Because it's such a small place, everybody was a caregiver," she said. "It was a really beautiful and unique model." Kirkpatrick worked hard to create dishes that the residents could enjoy, while also accompanying them through the death process. One patient with glioblastoma, an aggressive brain or spinal cord cancer, told Kirkpatrick that her worst fear was that her friends and family wouldn't be able to stay with her through the process as she died, that they would turn away. "For her husband, it created this amazing resolve," Kirkpatrick said, adding that he stayed present not only for her death, but also for the postmortem care and the transfer of the body to the morgue. "A lot of the things that you can see are very difficult to unsee." Kirkpatrick said that the guesthouse had a small elevator, meaning bodies strapped to a gurney had to be upended, causing them to shift in strange ways—and he stayed for all of that. "Stepping away is not a bad thing necessarily, but he had made that promise. And when he went to leave, he said, 'I feel that I did the best I could for her.' Which made his grief more bearable."

After patients were brought down the elevator and out into the garden, staff at the Guest House would open the bag down to the collarbone to display the patient laying on a pillow, and family gathered around. "Everybody would just basically say goodbye, and express gratitude for having had the opportunity to serve this person and this family," Kirkpatrick said. There would be bowls of rose petals, and family members and staff would sprinkle them on the body, while sometimes speaking words of farewell. Once, a volunteer whom Kirkpatrick had asked to sit with a body while waiting for the family to arrive shared something that moved her deeply. "What he said was that before today, I never had realized how much I could love somebody that I never knew," Kirkpatrick said. "And that was just the most beautiful thing. Because that's what would give you the energy to do that over and over again. That you can love someone so much that you've never even known."

Dieter sees the physician's role at the end of life as being to not run away, or state inaccurate phrases such as "there's nothing more I can do for you"—but rather, to show up authentically at the bedside. Over the years, he's learned how to do this better—partly through his studies with the Sacred Art of Living Center, an Oregon-based nonprofit offering workshops and professional development focused on whole-person caregiving. To stay grounded, Dieter posts something on Facebook every morning that he's grateful for, spends time in nature, and draws support from other members of the healthcare team. During weekly home care team meetings, staff will call out the name of each patient that's died while dropping a stone into a glass container; several times a year, they take these stones down to the shore of Lake Erie and hold a ceremony. And at the hospice house where Dieter works, staff gather on Monday and Thursday mornings in the meditation room, before the large windows overlooking the lake. They call out the name of each patient who's died since the previous meeting and ring a bell, then sit a few moments in reflection. Someone might share a song, a reading, or a poem. "It's just a way to ground ourselves, to remind ourselves of the work that we're doing and why we're there," Dieter said. "Ritual, in my experience, is tremendously helpful in doing self-care."

"Lightness and Depth at the Same Time"

Many hospice organizations and individual practitioners say rituals are an effective way for staff to honor patients who've died, to grieve, and to release the resulting emotions. Whether these ceremonies are organized as a hospice-wide or community event, engaged in by a particular healthcare team, or enacted in the privacy of one's home, they inevitably offer comfort, solace, and relief. One study suggests that they also heighten compassion and connection and prevent burnout.

Lisa Farmer, a kind woman with a grandmotherly manner who serves as the director of grief programs at Kansas City Hospice and Palliative Care, said that the organization has been holding its annual Circle of Lights memorial for over twenty years; typically, hundreds of people attend the outdoor event. There are usually about a thousand luminaries—votive candles nestled in sand inside a white bag—decorated with the person's name and punched with small holes for the light to come through. "We light them; they glow; dusk falls," Farmer said. While staff commonly request luminaries for a family member, attending the event allows them to reconnect with families they've served in the community, she said. "I think that's a very healing thing for our staff, to see these people that they made such an impact on and that are so grateful to see them. And that they're dressed, and they're out, and they're participating in communal events and observing the rituals of healing." Often, Farmer said, interdisciplinary healthcare teams will attend the event together, and have dinner beforehand. The event itself typically involves a responsive reading; a candle lighting ceremony; and a picture book about staying connected to a loved one, read while artists draw large scenes from the story in chalk. The ceremony concludes with a blessing and sending forth, during which people gather around their luminaries. Some bring flowers or other enhancements; many take them home.

Rituals that serve patients approaching death can also create an environment of peace and tranquility. Trish Rux, who worked as a nurse at a VA hospice in North Carolina for nearly ten years, often incorporated nonmedical modalities such as healing touch, mindfulness, and guided imagery to help her patients. For someone in intense pain, or who was waiting for the medication to take effect, she might put a hand on their heart or their back, while asking them questions about their pain: "Where are the edges to this? How big is it? What color is it? What's the texture? Where is it moving?" As a result, Rux said, patients would "get that sense that it's not as solid."

After becoming certified as a Sacred Passage Doula, Rux was inspired by an article she'd read to incorporate an anointing ritual, during which families—on their own, or led by a nurse or chaplain—would anoint a dying, or recently deceased, patient's body with lavender oil. Rux developed a script, and kept it simple so that families could incorporate other, more personal aspects. Lights were lowered, an LED candle was lit, and soft music played in the background as drops of oil were placed at different points on the body and family members bid farewell. "I noticed that not all of the people and their families had a faith tradition, and I felt there needed to be some way to mark and honor the sacredness," Rux said. "It gave them something special instead of, 'Your person died at 12:04, which funeral home do you want me to call?'" Rux said the ceremony also helped her let a patient go, while simple personal rituals such as showering, taking walks outside, meditating, or lighting a candle helped reduce the burnout from the cumulative impact of her work— she'd been at the bedside for at least 200 deaths. "There was definitely a conclusion aspect to it," she said of the ritual.

Lori Montross-Thomas, a psychologist, discovered the power of ritual when working in palliative care at San Diego Hospice. She'd noticed that a chaplain who'd been there more than twenty-five years—an elderly man with gray hair and a big smile—was always happy. Intrigued, she asked him what he did to making working in hospice a nourishing experience. The chaplain shared that over the years, he'd created leather-bound journals in which he'd write the first name of the patients he worked with, and every morning, he would place his hand on top of it and pray for them—for their passing, and for the continued health of their loved ones. That small act energized him for the day, he told her, and enabled him to truthfully say to patients that he kept them in his prayers. "I started thinking, I wonder if some of these seasoned clinicians have these kinds of rituals?" Montross-Thomas said, pointing out that while community ceremonies can be helpful, they happen only occasionally. "What do you do with all those other days when you've had a rough day, and you've had the death of a patient that you really cared about?"

Montross-Thomas undertook a national study asking hospice clinicians and volunteers about using rituals; to her surprise, 71 percent of respondents said they engaged in personal rituals, defined as "anything you do to personally honor your patients." Some attended funerals. Other common approaches included writing poems or journaling; saying a prayer; walking outdoors in the forest or at a beach; and picturing the deceased person while wishing them well. Clinicians said that the simplest rituals—things that could be easily enacted, without a lot of preparation—were most effective. Sometimes this meant opening a window with the intention of letting a patient's spirit pass. One clinician talked about sitting outside and letting the sun soak into her cells. Some identified rituals they hadn't even initially recognized, such as carefully handling paper documents related to a patient who'd died, perhaps while saying a blessing. Those who engaged in rituals reported significantly higher compassion satisfaction, as well as a lower burnout rating, when compared to those who didn't. When asked what they felt when doing a ritual, one clinician wrote: "A sense of lightness and depth at the same time."

Tabakin, the social worker at the New Jersey hospital system, said that she began seriously considering the power of rituals during the COVID-19 pandemic, when patients who'd recovered and were leaving the hospital were celebrated by playing a certain tone over the loudspeaker and people lining the halls to cheer them. "I just thought, 'Gosh, wouldn't it be nice if we actually gave that kind of attention and ritual to our deaths?'" she said. "It brings everything into more of a sacred space, and I think it's then more easily processed emotionally." Especially during the pandemic, Tabakin said, when there was so little ceremony or remembrance—often, not even a funeral—it felt essential to mark the importance of a person's life, even if she'd only known them for a few hours.

Because the clinicians were already so overworked and understaffed, Tabakin began to think about ways to help them identify rituals they were already doing. Often, clinicians feel pressured to engage in self-care and to develop coping mechanisms that only create an additional burden; telling staff to establish new rituals would be no different. "To all of us that just sounds like, 'Okay, here's another thing you're failing at, and you need to add something different into your life,'" Tabakin said. "Whereas this is about trying to identify what's already there and really turn that into the soil of nurturing." Sometimes staff would honor a veteran for their service, play music the patient enjoyed, or record the voices of their grandchildren to play for them. When Tabakin—who struggled with having to justify strict hospital visitation policies to families during the pandemic—had patients with COVID-19, she would hang a fabric butterfly on the doorknob to their room to remind herself to give those patients and families some extra attention. "We have one nurse who puts up these amazing cartoons in the staff bathroom, which bring so much joy and levity to people and are so meaningful," Tabakin said. "And then we have stones with encouraging words that we send with patients or family members."

For home hospice clinicians, such impromptu rituals are often performed in their cars as they move between patients. Montross-Thomas found that many would pull over to the side of the road and take a moment to reflect, cry, or listen to a specific song that they dedicated to the patient in their mind. Almerini, the home hospice nurse in New Jersey, said that she prefers to turn off the music and spend quiet time while driving. "I'll mostly seem to find my way to the ocean, because I live by the shore," she said. "So I'll make it a point to drive down by the ocean and either park there for a little while, or just contemplate it as I drive to the next patient." When she was working in an oncology unit as a young nurse, every time someone died, Almerini would stop at a nursery on the way home and buy a plant. "Now I have kind of a garden inside my house," she said. "It was the whole idea of just having something that was alive and living and growing."

On reflection, Montross-Thomas realized that she'd long performed a personal ritual that she hadn't identified as such. After a patient named Charlie died—one who Montross-Thomas had seen some thirty times on home visits, becoming close to him and his wife while getting to know their dogs and neighbors—she attended the funeral. Charlie's wife gave Montross-Thomas a silver votive candle holder in the shape of an angel, telling her that Charlie wanted her to have it because he always saw her as one of his Charlie's Angels. "It's so Charlie, because he was a bit cheeky," Montross-Thomas said. "I just thought, 'Oh, this is perfect.'" After that, every time Montross-Thomas lost a patient, she'd light a candle and let it burn through the night. "That was my vigil to them, and it was personalized," she said. "Other staff didn't know that I was doing it."

Montross-Thomas spent four years at San Diego Hospice; after it closed in 2013, she started a succulent design business—something unrelated to anything she'd done before. It was only once a friend of hers, a palliative care physician, pointed out that it made perfect sense that she saw a connection. "There was something invigorating about being with plants that were growing and blooming and you could design with them, and they were creating beauty in people's homes," said Montross-Thomas, who now teaches at the American University of the Caribbean School of Medicine in Sint Maarten. "So maybe all of us kind of have to figure out what is our threshold for how much we can take, and how much we need to monitor this sense of having a sense of grace and respect for the dying, but make sure we're also cultivating life for ourselves."

10

Palliative Care Forms Community

Alone we can do so little. Together we can do so much.

—HELEN KELLER

Emily Aaronson, an emergency physician and assistant chief quality officer at Massachusetts General Hospital, was working at the height of the COVID-19 surge when a ninety-eight-year-old patient came into her emergency department with the virus. The patient was short of breath and febrile, but relatively stable—at least initially. A goals-of-care conversation documented in her medical record several years prior had stated that the patient wanted a full code—CPR, intubation, and everything else. But when the palliative care team went to see her, they learned that the patient, who had metastatic cancer with underlying comorbidities, had actually spend the past year thinking about her life and the quality of her death and no longer wanted to be intubated. They were able to communicate this to the medical team, which felt much more supported in providing whole person care. "Things changed," Aaronson said, adding that the woman grew progressively worse and received comfort care before dying in the emergency department, according to her wishes. Without the conversations initiated by palliative care, "I worry that she would have been stuck on a vent and intubated in the ICU for weeks, and probably dying there," Aaronson said.

In recent years, palliative care teams have been key in assisting clinicians to navigate goals-of-care conversations with patients, while also addressing uncomfortable symptoms—such as pain, fatigue, and loss of appetite—for patients with serious illness. Thanks to technology, medical teams can now extend life much longer than was previously possible—advances that have even required the US to adopt a new definition of death. Prior to 1968, clinical death was defined as a cessation of heart and respiratory functions. But after the development of mechanical breathing machines and cardiac pacemakers in the mid-twentieth century, Harvard Medical School convened a committee to determine a new definition for death, one that included an irreversible loss of brain function. These developments led to the adoption of the Uniform Determination of Death Act in 1981, which defines death as "irreversible cessation of circulatory and respiratory functions" or "irreversible cessation of all functions of the entire brain."

While brain death is easily determined—it differs from minimally conscious or vegetative states in that there's no measurable brain activity—it's not impossible that it, too, may one day become reversible. "Whatever we consider irreversible by the standards of the time, that's what death is," said Christof Koch, chief scientist and president of the Allen Institute for Brain Science in Seattle. "So it used to be that heart and lung [function] were irreversible, but now that we can reverse that, it's the brain." Koch added that new research, in which scientists reactivated portions of pigs' brains four hours after their death, could one day call that definition into question. "We need a more rigorous scientific, mathematical, logical definition of death," he said.

While our current definition may be adequate for the capabilities of today's medical technology, it nevertheless leaves doctors to determine—along with patients, their families, and the rest of their medical team—when to accept that a patient is dying and to discontinue life-prolonging and often aggressive treatments. Increasingly, doctors are forced to hold difficult conversations around what it means to live and die well. When presented with the scenario of irreversible brain injury, most doctors would not choose any life-prolonging interventions for themselves—including CPR, feeding tubes, dialysis, and surgery, according to 1998 data from a decades-long study conducted at Johns Hopkins University. Yet helping patients to answer such questions for their own care is far more complicated, and requires a nuanced understanding of each individual's desires and goals for managing serious illness and end-of-life choices.

For Aaronson's ninety-eight-year-old patient, that meant revisiting a goals-of-care conversation in a critical moment. "I think she would have died either way," Aaronson said. "The question is, would she have died in the way that she wanted? And so I think that was a really amazing case where the team ended up feeling just so good about the care that they provided—that it was high quality, goal concordant, really appropriate care."

"Living as Well as Possible"

The term *palliative care* was coined in 1974 by Canadian surgical oncologist Balfour Mount as an alternative to hospice—which, in France, was a pejorative term associated with poor nursing home care that could be misconstrued by the French-speaking people in Montreal where he practiced. "The etymology was perfect," Mount said in an interview with McGill University, where he taught for over a decade. "It means to improve the quality of." While palliative care was initially established to address the needs of patients approaching the end of life, it has since evolved to provide comfort measures to patients with serious, life-limiting, or terminal illness early on in the disease process, and—unlike hospice—it can be combined with aggressive treatment measures such as chemotherapy or surgery.

Like many providers, Steven Pantilat, founding director of the palliative care program at the University of California, San Francisco (UCSF), has found the misconception that palliative care is only for the dying to be off-putting to patients who could benefit greatly from its services. "It's about how we help people with serious illness live as well as possible for as long as possible, recognizing that's going to be the likely experience for most of us—we're going to live longer, and we're going to live with serious illness," Pantilat said. Sometimes, this means managing physical symptoms such as pain, shortness of breath, and nausea. At others, it requires utilizing communication skills to help patients determine what's most important to them, the kind of care they would like to receive, and how they want to spend their remaining time—such as the patient with ALS who told Pantilat that he wanted to take a cruise with his wife; he'd never been on a cruise before. Pantilat told the patient that he should do so sooner rather than later, as he was only going to get weaker. "In palliative care, we don't shy away from that," he said. Palliative care provides patients with a range of support, including medical, practical, psychological, emotional, and spiritual. "That's why we practice as a team," Pantilat said. "We see patients together—as a nurse, social worker, chaplain, and physician—to be able to really address the variety of concerns that people have."

Access to palliative care has expanded considerably in recent years. In 2020, 72 percent of US hospitals containing more than fifty beds were found to house a palliative care team, a dramatic increase from the meager 7 percent reported in 2001. Pantilat, who also serves as director of UCSF's Palliative Care Leadership Center, which has helped more than two hundred hospitals establish programs nationwide, said the two biggest challenges to creating new teams are finding trained staff in the face of a workforce shortage and making the case to hire all of the team members despite the fact that only physicians—and sometimes other providers, such as nurse practitioners—can typically bill for insurance purposes. "The funding is by and large supported by institutions that see the benefit of it for their patients, and sometimes the financial benefit as well," Pantilat said. He added that once a new team is installed, they typically receive referrals very quickly. "Once we begin to provide the service there's a very quick uptake where people recognize the value," he said. Nevertheless, researchers are anticipating a growing workforce shortage as demand outpaces specialized clinicians in the relatively new field.

During the COVID-19 pandemic, palliative care expanded into areas of the hospital where there may have been less presence beforehand. "Palliative care virtually crashed into the emergency department nationwide," said Aaronson, who was the lead author on a research paper surveying 134 emergency department clinicians at her institution on their experiences with embedded palliative care during the pandemic. All of them indicated that they had experienced benefits as a result, such as being freed up to engage in other tasks, or feeling more supported. During weekly meetings, Aaronson said, both palliative care physicians embedded in the emergency department and emergency doctors benefiting from their services enthused about the impact they were having—including minimizing moral distress at the end of life. "In some cases, it's the patients for whom we provide very aggressive, invasive care and are not totally convinced that that's what the patient would have wanted, but we don't have the systems and support to sort of tease that out. And I think those are the shifts where people walk away with the moral distress of feeling like we didn't provide the patient with goal concordant care," Aaronson said. "And then there's the example on the other side, where we don't do everything because maybe there's a daughter or a family member [who advocated against it]; or we have a conversation with a patient, but it's not clear how skillful it is."

Despite palliative care's focus on quality of life, teams prove highly valuable to other clinicians when they're able to help patients and families discern end-of-life goals and desires. "I think it's important to begin those discussions relatively early on during a life-limiting illness, whether it's chronic or acute," said J. Randall Curtis, director of the Cambia Palliative Care Center of Excellence at the University of Washington. Curtis differentiates these conversations from advance directives—formal documents in which individuals can identify what sort of treatments they would—or wouldn't—want. Studies show only one-third of Americans have completed any kind of advance directive stating preferences for end-of-life care, including life-prolonging treatments such as intubation or CPR.

Curtis said that while these directives are not unimportant—especially in extreme situations such as that of Terri Schiavo, a woman in a persistent vegetative state whose husband and parents engaged in a prolonged court fight over whether or not to remove life support—they often don't clarify key aspects of future situations that may be hard to anticipate. Instead, Curtis advocates that younger or relatively healthy individuals establish a durable power of attorney for healthcare, or a healthcare surrogate, which identifies who they want to make decisions for them if they are incapacitated—an especially important move if this person is not their next-of-kin—and make sure that this person understands their values and can advocate on their behalf.

Other end-of-life documents, such as the Physician Order for Life-saving Treatments (POLST) or Medical Order for Life-Sustaining Treatment (MOLST) forms, are more applicable for those with chronic or terminal illness who can say that even in their current state, there would be certain kinds of treatment they wouldn't want, Curtis said. In such situations, having a directive on record can prevent highly undesirable or even traumatic outcomes for patients approaching the end of life. "One of the most stressful things for clinicians is trying to guide families through this when nobody really knows what the patient would want," Curtis said. "Patients themselves [often] choose less aggressive, less intensive care at the end of life than families choose for them. And this is a big source of distress for clinicians. They feel like they're providing care that families are requesting, that patients would not want."

Even providing goal-concordant care can sometimes place strain on clinicians. Tina Ha, a surgical oncology nurse at UCSF Mission Bay who's trained in palliative care, said that early on in her seven-year career, she would become upset when patients' family members pushed for more treatment, despite the fact that it was unlikely to extend the patient's life. But over time, she came to realize that everyone's ideas around death and dying are different. "Some patients just need to have that hope and option, and they need to know that they've tried everything," Ha said. "And just respecting that, even though that's not something I would want for myself or my family personally, it helped a lot. It helped me do my job, because we're the ones administering all these treatments, and if you feel like you disagree with them, you feel like it's wrong, it's definitely going to affect you and make you feel like a horrible person." Ha said that although she initially felt unable to display her feelings in front of patients, she also learned that it was okay to do so—particularly after taking an eight-week compassion training. "It's really just being present with the patient and not saying things like, 'Oh it will be OK,'" she said. "Because I feel like in healthcare we always feel like we have to offer a solution or a remedy. But sometimes there's just not." Meanwhile, connecting with chaplains and social workers on the palliative care team enabled her to unload some of her struggles. She attended the patient memorial events held every six months, while finding personal ways to commemorate patients she'd lost, such as dedicating her yoga practice to a patient who'd loved yoga and had died when her daughter was pregnant. "I think about her from time to time, and about the family, and hope they're doing well," Ha said.

Members of palliative care teams often provide essential support to each other, as well as to physicians, nurses, and other healthcare staff managing difficult emotions around grief and trauma. "Our experience caring for really sick people, and people who die, gives us some insight into how to approach it and how to deal with it," Pantilat said. "So we do help our colleagues deal with these really difficult and challenging situations." Pantilat emphasized that the inclusion of chaplains and social workers on palliative care teams is essential to meeting the needs of both staff and patients. "It definitely helps to prevent burnout," he said of the team model, adding that a chaplain at UCSF has developed a series of self-care trainings. The hospital has also implemented Schwartz Rounds, which provide a forum for clinicians to decompress and discuss the emotional, rather than the clinical, aspects of a case. As chief of the division, Pantilat said he also strives to create schedules and work hours that promote sustainability and resilience. "There's no point in having people overwork and burn out and leave," he said.

"Treated with Dignity and Respect"

Despite the recent expansion and heightened availability of palliative care, many states and populations remain severely underserved. While palliative care is widely available in the US northeast and mountain regions, it remains limited in south-central states, as well as in rural areas, where only 17 percent of hospitals with fifty beds or more report palliative care teams. Meanwhile, minorities face significant barriers to obtaining hospice and palliative care. The vast majority of hospice recipients are white, while minorities utilize their services at rates far below their representation in the general population. Dulce Cruz-Oliver, a geriatrician and internist who teaches at Johns Hopkins Medicine and has worked as medical director of both a nursing home and a hospice company, was inspired to study the lack of knowledge around end-of-life options for Latino patients and their caregivers. She said some of it is as simple as resolving misunderstandings: many Latinos' interpretation of the word *hospicio*, for example, is as an orphanage—the last place they would want to leave their loved ones. Other approaches involved exploring ways for Latinos to overcome restrictions to getting professional help, which would allow them to keep their dying family member longer at home. After doing interviews and focus groups with Latino patients and caregivers about what they wanted, Cruz-Oliver surveyed hospice staff on how to best educate them and—based on these suggestions—created a telenovela called *Cuidadores Como Yo* (*Caregivers Like Me*). Cruz-Oliver said she thinks that many of her patients and their families are affected by a decision not to enroll in hospice. "But for me, quality end-of-life care, it's not the same as the patient in front of me," she said. "For some people, quality of dying is to die in the ICU. For other people it's not, they prefer not to be surrounded by tubes. And that's fine—it's just, people are different." While limited research has been conducted on the disparities within palliative care, a study published by the *Journal of American Society of Nephrology* shed light on how Black and Hispanic dialysis patients from 2006 through 2014 were significantly less likely to receive palliative care services inside the hospital when compared to white dialysis patients.

Clinicians bringing palliative care to disenfranchised areas or populations must develop additional communication skills, advocate for resources, and push for education around cultural understanding—often without the support and backup provided by a full palliative care team. Karen Bullock, a palliative care researcher with sleek, black hair and high cheekbones who heads the School of Social Work at North Carolina State University and has spent decades doing clinical social work in inpatient and outpatient settings, said that some of her greatest difficulties as a palliative care provider involved getting clinicians to see things through a cultural lens for Black patients and family members. With her own mother—who, after being diagnosed with stage four metastatic lung cancer, decided against hospice—Bullock found herself highly offended when the radiation oncologist had trouble accepting her mother's choice to decline further treatment. "I'll always remember sitting in the room with this physician," Bullock said. "And she said to me, 'I don't think your mother is understanding what I'm saying.'" The physician was advocating the potential to extend her mother's life by five years or more, but it wasn't what her mother wanted. "The challenging part is to get medical teams to see a patient who's different than the typical patient that they usually see and to think about the fact that this patient or this family might actually have strengths," Bullock said. "The way in which they function might actually be serving them very well. And there might be good reasons why they don't want to do this, and they will feel better emotionally, psychologically, and otherwise when they know that their wishes are being honored and they're being treated with dignity and respect."

Bullock connected with Black and brown families at the end of life who had long been disenfranchised by the medical system, many of whom were religious. Sometimes, a patient would be brain dead, but because they looked the same, the family believed there was still a possibility for recovery. Once, a family told her that they believed in miracles, and that they were waiting on the Lord. "I understand that language," said Bullock, who grew up in a Black Baptist church. "So I said to them, 'Well, while you're waiting on the Lord, can we consider a few other things?' And so they start to listen differently than they had been listening—or not listening—previously, because I was able to speak their language."

Bullock said that the approach of palliative care teams often runs counter to Black and brown people's values—such as speaking to the patient alone, without family members present—while the notion of advanced care planning often seems irrelevant to those who don't have many assets or who count on family members to handle hard decisions. "It's inconsistent culturally with the way we're socialized and acculturated," Bullock said. "And it all is related to systemic racism. If we look at the culture of people of color in this country, we know there were good reasons for people not to divulge information and not to share information. We also know that structurally people of color weren't allowed to access these care settings. And so now that they can, the care providers expect people of color to be like, 'Yay, we're so happy. And we trust these people.' They're still not trusting of this type of care. They feel like, 'Okay, so you want me to have a good quality of life now that I'm dying?'" Bullock would like to see hospitals establish measurable standards for cultural competency while recognizing and naming the role of systemic racism.

For other communities, palliative care remains completely inaccessible. Mary Isaacson, an associate professor at South Dakota State University College of Nursing and former hospice coordinator, said that access to palliative care is limited in the state's rural areas. Meanwhile, it doesn't exist in Indian Health Service (IHS) facilities, which serve eight reservations in South Dakota, at all. In 2018, Isaacson published a qualitative study in the *International Journal of Palliative Nursing* based on talking circles involving elders and tribal health educators in an attempt to understand perceptions of palliative care within their community. She discovered that participants found the basic principles culturally congruent with their life philosophies, though none of them had heard of hospice or palliative care before. They also stated that IHS personnel seeking to implement such services would need cultural awareness training as well as the ability to speak and understand relevant languages. Moreover, participants recognized the challenges posed by geography, a general lack of services, and minimal financial support.

Health services on the reservations in general are lacking, and the IHS is severely underfunded. While under the Affordable Care Act (ACA), the Indian Health Care Improvement Act (IHCIA) authorized hospice, assisted living, and other forms of elder care, there's not enough money for even basic services. Other issues include high turnover, making it difficult for individuals to establish long-term relationships with a primary care provider, and cultural misunderstanding and miscommunication. "One thing if you're going to be talking about difficult news, or before beginning an exam or something, is offering a prayer before you do so you start in the right way," Isaacson said. "And if you look at our healthcare system, how many of us are willing to do that?" Isaacson is now working on a grant to develop culturally appropriate messaging, drawing on the success of an earlier program in which tribal elders educated community members about advance directives. "When you think about a messaging campaign, that is who is a trusted and respected member of the community, who should be delivering this message about palliative and end-of-life care," she said. "It was Native to Native; it was person to person; community member to community member."

Tinka Duran, the prevention programs director at the Great Plains Tribal Leaders Health Board and an enrolled member of the Rosebud Sioux Tribe who's been assisting Isaacson to develop these initiatives, said the lack of palliative care is a serious issue. Duran, who oversees eight different programs focusing mostly on cancer prevention and screening, said she noted early on in her fourteen years with the health board the impact of the lack of palliative care on cancer patients. "Even with diabetes, when my grandmother was dying and not being able to get comfort care, or hospice care," Duran said, "there's none of that as well in our tribal communities. So we really relied on the family to help with bathing and all those types of daily things that people take for granted." Meanwhile, lack of cultural competency means that providers may not understand concepts such as using traditional healers and ceremonies at the end of life, or the meaning of *wakunza*—which suggests that talking about something might bring it on. To better understand the communities in which they work, Duran suggests that providers simply ask in a respectful manner and allow time for elders, who may take a long pause before speaking, to be heard.

In order to obtain the care they need, Duran said, many individuals end up leaving the reservation at the end of life. "Many of our people end up dying alone because the family doesn't have the resources or places to stay up in those communities or those big cities," she said. Others aren't even able to make it off the reservations themselves. "Our people live on dirt roads, there may not be any gravel," she said. "And if it rains, they're not getting out. If it snows, you know, they may not be getting out. The reality is that poverty is a big factor. Many of our people, to meet their basic needs, are trying to figure out if I have enough gas to get to palliative care services, versus going to get groceries, which one am I going to do first? They're probably going to go get groceries."

Duran said that while it can be hard to witness the struggles suffered by her people, it also makes her motivated to try even harder. "It just hits you right here in the heart, just to see our people suffering," she said. "Not being able to get those resources or care—it's painful. It hurts, you know? And sometimes you cry." Once, Duran found herself suffering from *wakunza* herself when she began to feel like every ache or pain was cancer, but she saw a traditional healer who told her that this work was what she was supposed to be doing. "That relieved a lot of it and of course made me even more dedicated," said Duran, who goes for walks and attends ceremonies to take care of herself. "You're going to get discouraged, but you've just got to keep going, because you know what you're doing is for the good of the whole community."

Duran said that telehealth and transportation support are vital necessities, as is more education and federal funding for healthcare initiatives—often, she said, available funding is established along expedited timelines that work for corporations and larger hospitals, but not for tribal organizations that need to obtain approval from the tribal government or retain ownership over data. Many organizations have been using telehealth effectively: Pantilat at UCSF said that even prior to the COVID-19 pandemic, over half the division's visits were through telemedicine, serving patients who live farther away or those too sick to come in, while sometimes including family members across the country. Meanwhile, Medicare began covering telehealth visits more broadly during the COVID-19 pandemic—allowing clinicians such as Susan McCammon, a head and neck surgeon and professor at the University of Alabama at

Birmingham who provides palliative care both to her surgical cancer patients and within the community at large, to switch largely to tele-health. "The number of times that I asked somebody to show me their wound and they showed me their ceiling fan," McCammon said, laughing. "It's not perfect, but it really broadens our access." McCammon has found the medium to be a real boon to reaching patients in Alabama, where all sixty-seven counties have rural areas—prior to the pandemic, she had been providing palliative care to ambulatory patients in clinic and doing more home visits, in addition to offering telehealth in more rural areas. "So much of palliative care is talk-based that I find having a telehealth or a home-based visit is equally effective," she said.

McCammon said that she'd learned a lot from the research her colleague, Ronit Elk, had done on cultural respect and competency with the African-American and rural white populations in Alabama. "A couple of the things that she's really identified are the need for inclusion of family and pastoral care in decision-making," McCammon said. "I've had several patient encounters where the pastor has been a crucial intermediary in helping manage expectations and treatment decisions. And that's not something that I normally would gravitate toward, but now I do." Now, McCammon asks all of her patients if there's someone else they'd like involved in their decision-making process. She's also learned to better express humility—including the possibility of miracles. "When I have patients who are hoping for a miracle, part of what I do is I say, 'You know, I'm hoping for this miracle with you, but while we're hoping for that miracle, let's prepare for if it doesn't happen.'" McCammon recently shared these words with a patient with a bad prognosis. "She just broke down and said, 'No physician has ever said that to me before. No one has ever said that a miracle might be possible,'" McCammon said. "For her, it was an incredibly powerful statement for a physician to cede their authority and say, 'You know what, I don't really know what's going to happen here.'"

Palliative care practitioners in underserved areas are uniquely challenged by the fact that they have little support; few resources; and are navigating cultural differences that are not always well understood by medical providers. Meanwhile, they are already on the outskirts of a relatively new profession with a significant workforce shortage—one that is only expected to worsen as the aging population grows. While many researchers advocate basic palliative care training for primary care physicians as a way to improve access, this approach is also not ideal, as it would remove the support provided by a team with multiple practitioners. And McCammon, for one, has come to realize the value of having separate providers. "One of the things I've seen is that patients feel apprehensive about expressing doubt or weakness in front of their primary treating physician, whether it's an oncologist or a surgeon," McCammon said. "So having the opportunity to have a second pair of eyes or a neutral ear is really important."

"Taking the Long Lens"

Considering the strain on palliative care providers and the uniquely challenging circumstances they encounter, one might imagine they experience more burnout—but the data is not so clear. In 2016, Arif Kamal, a medical oncologist and palliative medicine specialist at Duke Cancer Center and associate professor at Duke University School of Medicine, was the lead author on a paper finding that palliative care clinicians experienced much more widespread burnout when compared to their colleagues in other specialties. However, when conducting a similar study two years later, he learned their original calculations had been erroneous, requiring them to retract the previous document. Instead, palliative care clinicians reported burnout at rates essentially comparable to other clinicians. "Both findings were surprising to me," said Kamal, who had received a lot of feedback from palliative care clinicians that the earlier results made sense. "I worry that the message may be that we're just in line with everybody else. And actually I think a lot about the workforce itself, and why there probably are some nuances to that data." Roughly half of physicians providing palliative care have chosen it as a second career, which means they could simply be retiring rather than reporting burnout, while palliative care clinicians often have mixed careers with other specialties such as family medicine, Kamal said. Meanwhile, he's received feedback from some palliative care physicians that they thought burnout would be relatively lower in their field, because they were more accustomed to encountering suffering and distress.

Palliative care social workers and nurses reported higher rates of burnout than physicians—which Kamal attributes to the fact that doctors have more opportunity to step away for continuing education, attending conferences, or teaching; his qualitative research has backed this assertion. "Physicians are more likely to have no two days that are alike; that includes a lot of unique opportunities to do things other than face-to-face clinical care," he said. "Physicians, too, are the ones who have diverse practices, so they may see their outpatient clinic in the morning and then go do palliative care consults in the afternoon. And so I think that sort of role variation is very helpful." Nurses and social workers immersed in direct patient care, meanwhile, have little-to-no break from ongoing encounters with those who are seriously ill, suffering, and dying.

As the American population ages, placing greater strain on the workforce, Kamal's research predicts that palliative care physicians could be expected to see twenty or more patients daily, as opposed to the current standard of eight to ten patients—further contributing to burnout. "We start to worry about issues not only about safety and quality of care, certainly, but also the emotional resilience of the workforce to provide that, because it's really hard," he said. "One of the reasons why palliative care can be very rewarding is that you get time with patients—because you're sort of a witness to their distress and you're able to give them techniques and talk them through it. As that goes down, potentially due to some pressures from payers and regulators and so on, it starts to introduce potentially some moral injury as well, which is this injury of over promising and under delivering." In addition, financial pressures on a team that force them to exclude necessary members such as a social worker or chaplain could create moral injury by reducing a doctor's ability to provide the holistic care they're promising, Kamal said, adding: "I think the field right now is starting to see some early components of that."

Kamal noted one time when he would have benefited from the presence of a larger team: he was seeing a 60-year-old woman with advanced
ovarian cancer who was experiencing significant abdominal pain. Kamal
spent a half-hour discussing how she could manage her pain with opioids
and making sure she understood the potential side effects. When she
returned two weeks later, Kamal asked, in his usual gentle manner, how
her pain was—and she said it was still a ten out of ten. "I thought this
was a medical problem, because I'm a medical doctor," Kamal said. He
counseled her further to make sure that she understood, and sent her
on her way. Two weeks later, her pain was still a ten out of ten. Finally,
Kamal performed a very basic spiritual assessment during which he discovered that the woman believed that because she'd had an abortion
in her teenage years, the ovarian cancer was God's punishment and the
pain was part of her atonement. "She actually needed an intervention
from somebody who could kind of talk her through that, because she was
debilitated by pain and in tears, yet at the same time trying to balance
these two things," Kamal said. "If I had, for example, included a chaplain
in that multidisciplinary care from the very beginning that person would
likely have caught that before I did and been able to address that."

In addition to chaplains, Kamal has found social workers incredibly
valuable because they've been trained in a different way. "They have
supervisors who follow their practice with whom they debrief one-on-
one, not about the management components or the patient care components," he said. "But the 'How are you doing with this? How are you
holding someone else's distress and still able to go home and hug your
kids? And how is that affecting you? What are the issues of transference
and countertransference?' And I think that's a really important model
for palliative medicine." At Duke, Kamal said, the palliative care social
workers have trained some other members of the team to hold regular
debriefings during which they discuss why it's hard to take care of patients
with serious illness. "The purpose of the discussion is not to arrive at a fix,
it's to hear each other and normalize it and say yes, we're all struggling,"
he said. "And there is some solace in not feeling alone." Kamal noted
that this can be especially important for palliative care clinicians, who

work within a culture of heroism due to the specialty's foundation as a grassroots movement to correct the injustice of bad care for patients with advanced and serious illness. "The challenge with that, obviously, is that you can become a martyr to the cause, and that's a slippery slope," Kamal said. "Because you see so much injustice and you see so much need. And so then you can start to sacrifice your own mental health and energy." One small, personal action that Kamal takes to care for his own well-being—especially during the COVID-19 pandemic, when he was more often providing telehealth from home—is to create a ritual to separate work from the rest of his life. "I ritually may leave the house either to drive around the block or to walk around the house and sort of switch into home mode from that," he said.

Still, Kamal emphasized that beyond personal measures and debriefings, there are systemic issues at play that must be addressed. "If I'm writing my notes at home at nine o'clock at night after seeing all my patients, well, that's not helpful," he said. "Or if the system doesn't reward seeing lots of patients, or if there's no autonomy in scheduling, for example, so people are constantly working on their kids' birthdays. There are things like that that are actually quite system-level that frankly yoga and meditation, other things, are not going to overcome." Another issue Kamal identified is that palliative care teams are often brought in as consultants but not empowered to write orders for pain medication or other things they recommend. "That's one of those things where you feel very invested in how someone's care should change or be different, but you can't actually make it happen," he said. "That starts to wear on people, too."

Toward the beginning of the COVID-19 pandemic, Stacie Sinclair, the associate director for policy at the Center to Advance Palliative Care (CPAC) based at the Icahn School of Medicine at Mount Sinai in New York City, authored a blog on burnout for palliative care physicians—and it quickly became the most popular post of the year. Individual level approaches that she said have helped include peer support systems—such as buddy systems, in which clinicians are paired with another individual in their workplace who really understands the environment—in addition to mental health treatment, mindfulness-based stress reduction, mentorship, and physician wellness coaching. "It's a place to turn to if it's just a really bad situation or a bad day," Sinclair said of the buddy system. "And really, that goes that much further when the team or the department lead is institutionalizing the program. . . . I think that having that support from the top can be really helpful."

Like Kamal, Sinclair recognized that there is only so much that can be done at the individual level. "You need to be operating in a system that truly supports wellness," she said. "So what resources is your organization making available to you? Do you have the therapy services? Do you have enough capacity to be able to take time off if you really need the time? Are there clear boundaries around working hours? At a practical level, is the healthcare coverage that you're giving—your insurance—does it cover the necessary services that folks need to be able to pursue their own mental health?"

Rev. Paula Teague, the senior director of spiritual care and chaplaincy for the Johns Hopkins Health System and a Society of Friends (Quaker) minister, said that while chaplains commonly experience a feeling of being stretched too thinly, the hospital where she oversees chaplaincy services, Johns Hopkins Bayview Medical Center, has some per diem chaplains that allow the regular staff to take time off when necessary. "If we're wounded, we're not going to be able to really help other people very much," Teague said. "So there's got to be that attention to having time off and some self-care time, too." During the COVID-19 pandemic, chaplains were at the bedside when families often weren't able to be, she said. Sometimes, they'd comfort family members afterward—such as the distraught husband who'd come into the hospital shortly after his wife had died, upset that their last words on the telephone had been an argument. "We sat with him and helped him to say to her now what he would like to have said before she died," Teague said. "And I think it gave him some comfort, to understand that she could hopefully still hear him."

Teague said that in addition to participating in goals-of-care conversations and providing spiritual care to patients and family members, chaplains—whether on a palliative care team or not—do a great deal of staff and provider support. "We help staff, and we do staff huddles and try to provide inspiration, hope," she said. "Really help people build resilience." That support system works both ways, Teague said. Once, she'd stepped away from a conversation with someone who'd lost a family member to suicide—not recently, but in the past—and was feeling very tired. She got into the elevator with one of the doctors she often worked with, and he noted that she didn't look well. "I said, 'I'm really disturbed by this conversation I had,'" Teague said. "And you know, he got off the elevator with me at the floor where I was going, and sat there and talked to me for a few minutes about it. I thanked him later—it struck me later how caring that was. Just in the moment, to have somebody say, 'Gosh, Paula, you don't look like you're doing so great right this minute.' So I think there's a lot of mutuality there, and a lot of teamwork and respect, and I think that goes a long way."

Palliative care clinicians have repeatedly identified debriefings as an effective means of processing emotions. About a year into the pandemic, the CAPC began offering a training on providing wellness debriefings, a structure developed by social worker Victoria Leff to give healthcare professionals a space in which to reflect on their experiences and normalize what they're going through. "It can be topic driven; it can be open-ended," Sinclair said, adding that debriefings provide essential support by "creating a safe space in a group, to bring people together and just take some time to pause, and be able to express: What are some of the challenges that you're facing?" Sinclair said that while some institutions have accepted the need for such measures, others require further education on why it's worth dedicating staff time and resources. "I think part of it is taking the long lens," she said. "Healthcare providers are starting to understand that there are real consequences to not caring for your workforce, particularly in heightened circumstances like COVID has created."

John Wax, a palliative care physician at the University of Vermont Medical Center, said that he has been working with colleagues in pediatrics to develop curriculum for debriefing patient deaths. They started the program in early 2019 after some pediatric residents, who'd experienced a number of difficult oncology deaths, expressed in their annual wellness survey that this had led to depression, isolation, and a heightened sense of imposter syndrome. "They couldn't help, they couldn't fix the problem," Wax said. They were "sort of wondering if they did the right things, or could it have been less traumatic in some way, or were certain things said that were unhelpful." While the debriefings initially focused on residents, nurses soon began to express interest in participating, and they decided to expand it to everybody who'd had direct experience with the patient— including primary care physicians, hospice nurses, licensed nursing assistants, interpreters, child life specialists, social workers, chaplains, and others. Somewhere from eight to twenty-four participants typically attend; after the COVID-pandemic began and the conversations moved to Zoom, their reach expanded—once including a doctor in Boston. "Sometimes the conclusions at the end of the meetings are like, 'It's okay to be raw. It's okay to swear,'" Wax said, adding that it's important for clinicians "to share stories of compassion, or joy sometimes, before or around the time of dying, and also to help everybody weave a full narrative together." Many may not have encountered their patients when they were active—or even fully conscious—and sometimes, clinicians can flesh out this picture for one another, such as the nurse who'd previously served as a camp counselor for a pediatric patient. "Otherwise the hospital feels like an assembly line," Wax said. "If you don't have the context of who that person is, then you're actually just treating disease, you're not treating a person. And we often don't have enough time to pause."

While palliative care clinicians are embracing debriefings and other methods to address burnout, their growing presence in areas such as the emergency department and intensive care unit often proves support to other clinicians, particularly in regards to the moral distress associated with end-of-life care. May Hua, an assistant professor of anesthesiology at Columbia University who has studied the impact of palliative care in the ICU, found that patients in hospitals involved in palliative care programs were 46 percent more likely to be discharged into hospice, as opposed to those without. "Hospice is generally viewed as a desirable outcome," Hua said. "Their symptoms are very cared for, grieving is better in caregivers, they get rehospitalized less, they have less medicalized deaths—which, again, tends to go more in line with what people say they want." On a personal level, Hua has found palliative care clinicians to be particularly helpful for patients in her ICU who are there for longer periods, because their staffing model means that the attending physicians switch out each week. "It's actually more important to have somebody there who's really asking that question [about the direction of care], making sure that more bird's-eye view is being considered," she said.

Healthcare workers are greatly comforted by knowing that they're providing the care a patient would have wanted, and by having family members on board with the decision. Palliative care teams are often essential to achieving such outcomes and preventing moral injury—particularly in the ICU and ER, where clinicians are often stretched thin and don't have time to engage in lengthy conversations. While a lack of cultural competency and access for rural and underserved populations has created significant challenges for clinicians seeking to make inroads in these areas, all palliative care team members are affected by the specialty's workforce shortage and lack of resources. Healthcare organizations willing to invest in robust palliative care teams inevitably provide much better care—not only to patients, but also to the wider community of physicians, nurses, and other clinical staff.

11

Assisted Dying Brings Comfort and Concern

Think occasionally of the suffering of which you spare yourself the sight.

—ALBERT SCHWEITZER

Terminally ill patients who feel that hospice and palliative care are not sufficient to address their physical anguish or declining abilities will sometimes ask clinicians to help them die—an option that has only recently become legal in some states, and can cause significant moral distress for clinicians, while creating legal and professional ramifications. Timothy Quill, a palliative care physician and professor emeritus at the University of Rochester Medical Center, had helped many patients to navigate difficult end-of-life issues when he met a patient he called "Diane," with acute myelomonocytic leukemia, in the late 1980s. She refused chemotherapy and enrolled in home hospice, and while Quill had some initial misgivings about her choice, he came to understand her desire to avoid the side effects of chemotherapy and hospitalization. Yet Diane wanted more: she feared a lingering death, and so Quill referred her to a right-to-die organization called the Hemlock Society. And when Diane requested barbiturates for sleep, an essential ingredient for the method of suicide outlined by the society, Quill agreed—informing her of the proper amounts for both sleep and suicide. "I wrote the prescription with an uneasy feeling about the boundaries I was exploring—spiritual, legal, professional, and personal," Quill later wrote of the case in the *New England Journal of Medicine.* "Yet I also felt strongly that I was setting her free to get the most out of the time she had left, and to maintain dignity and control on her own terms until her death." As her level of pain, discomfort, and dependence increased, Diane bid farewell to family, friends—and to Quill—and took the medication. Quill, who'd taken a significant risk to prescribe it at a time when assisted dying was illegal everywhere in the US, then took an even greater gamble: he went public with her story.

Quill, who had discussed the move with trusted colleagues beforehand, felt it was important to get the issue out in the open. At the time, Jack Kevorkian, an outlier popularly known as "Dr. Death" who advocated for medical experiments on death row inmates and the creation of suicide clinics, had taken hold of the public imagination by assisting in more than one hundred deaths—one of which resulted in a second-degree murder verdict. "I thought about my experience with Diane, and said, 'Well, you know, I'm a pretty mainstream person,'" Quill said. "And this is potentially a pretty mainstream idea. It got marginalized because of Kevorkian in many ways. So I thought it'd be a lot harder to dismiss and might get the conversation going at a deeper level." While Quill anticipated some backlash, he was unprepared for the breadth of the impact—including national media attention, investigations, and a potential criminal indictment that was eventually declined by a grand jury. Later, Quill became the lead plaintiff in a case challenging the constitutionality of New York's ban on physician-assisted suicide; the US Supreme Court decided in 1997 that the ban was, in fact, constitutional.

Yet Quill's advocacy had significant impact on the national debate, which has, in recent decades, become much more amenable to what is commonly known as medical aid in dying (MAID). Since Oregon passed its Death with Dignity Act in 1997, the practice has become legal in eight other states and Washington, DC—most recently in New Mexico, where it was signed into law in April 2021—while others are considering legislation. While each state law differs slightly (e.g., it's legal in Montana due to a state Supreme Court ruling rather than a statute), the requirements are generally stringent. Patients must have a terminal illness with a diagnosis of less than six months to live; approval from two physicians, one of whom prescribes the lethal dose of medication; be of sound mind; and have the ability to ingest the medication themselves. This final requirement differentiates the practice from active euthanasia in which lethal medication is administered by a physician. Physician-administered euthanasia remains illegal across the US—meaning those seeking MAID don't qualify if they're unable to self-administer—potentially protecting patients from abuse. In contrast, physician-administered euthanasia is legal in the Netherlands, though informed and conscious consent is required.

The moral and ethical implications of MAID place significant strain on clinicians, who must navigate the related—and often thorny—professional and legal issues. The question is literally one of life or death. Whether they support MAID or find it abhorrent, doctors are forced to evaluate their most deeply held beliefs and professional stances—ones that may not always align with the current legal framework. Some, like Quill, take significant risks to do what they feel will best support their patients. Others find themselves questioning whether their chosen profession has forgotten its purpose. Meanwhile, nurses, chaplains, and others at the bedside are burdened with figuring out how to best support patients while also adhering to strict rules and procedures, and seeking out scarce educational platforms, tools, and resources or relying on inadequate information. Clinicians on both sides of the debate, whether they are involved in the process or not, have struggled to align the legal status of the issue with their personal ethics, professional obligations, and moral beliefs.

"A Terrible Position to Be In"

Even in states where aid in dying is legal, there can be significant barriers, as Barbara Morris, a geriatric advocate and doctor in Colorado, discovered when a patient named Neil Mahoney approached her for help. Mahoney, who had recently been diagnosed with a painful form of glandular cancer that had spread to his liver and beyond, was struggling through chemotherapy. He'd been given less than six months to live, and was seeking aid in dying under Colorado's End-of-Life Options Act. But because Morris worked for Centura Health Corporation—a Christian system that had opted out of providing the service—she was unable to meet his request. "It's a terrible position to be in," Morris said. She felt the moral distress of abandoning her patient at a critical point on his journey. "To be prevented from providing a patient with something that is a legal medical procedure, being told you can't do that, is actually horrifying."

Morris began to question the difference between Centura's policy, which forbade participation in aid in dying, and the Colorado statute, which said that health systems can opt out for patients planning to use it on their premises. Mahoney didn't fit that category—he had hoped to take the medication at home. In August 2019, the two of them filed a legal complaint seeking to prevent Centura from prohibiting Morris from prescribing the medication. A few days later, Centura fired Morris. "Not only did that interrupt my ability to care for Neil, but it interrupted my ability to care for hundreds of other patients," said Morris, who had worked with some of them for many years and placed great value on providing continuous care. "It was as bad as it could get."

Mahoney eventually managed to obtain aid in dying from a pharmacist, while Morris amended the lawsuit to employment-related claims including wrongful discharge; as of early 2021, the legal process was ongoing. "I was relieved, of course," Morris said of Mahoney's ability to access the medication. "It really highlighted, though, how challenging the situation can be in Colorado, even though we have a statute. There are still so many barriers and so many hurdles for patients and their families." (The once commonly used barbiturates can now cost more than $3,000 and aren't always covered by insurance, causing doctors to seek other options, while those in rural areas can have trouble accessing amenable physicians, among other challenges.) Morris, meanwhile, took some time to figure out her next steps, and in February 2020 accepted a job at a health center in Denver. The lawsuit and loss of her job "totally threw my entire life into disarray," she said. "It was a complete mess, a complete nightmare, not one I had ever anticipated having to go through."

Thalia DeWolf, a hospice nurse and board member for the American Clinicians Academy on Medical Aid in Dying (ACAMAID), said that when the California law first took effect in 2016, hospice administrators and clinicians were commonly fearful of professional or legal repercussions—and that many remain so today. When her patient, who had a neurogenerative disease and did not want a prolonged death, was the first to take medical aid in dying at her Northern California hospice that year, DeWolf was terrified she would get fired. "There was so much information about what I was not allowed to do, and not a lot of information about how to really support the patient," DeWolf said. DeWolf was required to leave the room at the moment of ingestion—not by law, but due to hospice policy based on fear of litigation—which created moral distress by making her feel like she was abandoning her charge. "I had one arm around the patient's daughter who was weeping on my shoulder; I had one hand on the foot of the patient," she said about the day of ingestion. "I had to what I call 'pop that sacred bubble' and walk out the room. It was amongst the most embarrassing and terrible things I think I've ever done." While some nurses prefer to leave the room to give the family privacy, DeWolf said, most families want clinicians to remain present. "That first moment after ingestion is traumatic," she said. "It's hard for families."

Not long after the California statute passed, Lonny Shavelson, a longtime advocate for aid in dying, opened his own clinic—Bay Area End of Life Options—and invited DeWolf to join him. For the next four years, DeWolf was at the bedside of roughly one hundred patients as they underwent the procedure. She would ensure that they were also receiving hospice and palliative care, and was comforted by the fact that she was able to be present when they died. She said that MAID deaths differ from other deaths in that they happen quickly—typically in one to four hours, as opposed to over days or weeks—and that patients can develop agonal breathing, a brainstem reflex that sounds like a mixture of a gasp and a groan, or their lips can turn blue. Being present allowed her to assure families that the patient was completely unconscious, and that this was normal. In 2020, they closed the practice because, DeWolf said, "we were becoming the Planned Parenthood of aid in dying and we didn't want to"—meaning that people were becoming overly reliant on their services, rather than developing their own practices. Now, the two of them cooperate on ACAMAID, a nonprofit that both patients and clinicians can use as a resource for referrals, educational videos, and other tools.

DeWolf has shared much of her knowledge on the platform, including how to mix the medications, what to expect with an aid in dying death, and other key considerations. "I'm probably amongst a very few number of nurses in the country who've been able to really support patients through medical aid in dying," DeWolf said. "Often in hospice, they're not barred, but they're just hobbled." Many institutions have a "don't ask, don't tell policy," which breeds shame; nurses are often prohibited from mentioning the subject unless a patient uses obvious and explicit language; and relevant nursing education is sorely lacking, DeWolf said—despite the necessity of monitoring patients in the weeks prior to the procedure to ensure they're swallowing and not suffering from nausea, and the somewhat complicated nature of mixing the medications. At her current hospice, DeWolf finds that often, neither the hospice doctors nor the doctor who's prescribed the medication want to take responsibility for those final weeks of life, while families lose out when medical staff is not present for the death event—a common occurrence she believes is fueled by fear of repercussions. In essence, many practitioners involved in MAID feel forced to erect a wall between themselves and their patients, which can create a greater sense of depersonalization and alienation for patients and families as well as providers. "I had one family who did it on their own and later reported to me that they felt like it was like an Ikea death," DeWolf said. "They had just followed the instructions, because it was complex, and they weren't there emotionally."

An analysis of the data from Oregon and Washington between MAID's legal debut and 2017, published in *JAMA Network Open*, found that a total of 3,368 prescriptions were written for patients, with 76 percent dying from lethal ingestion. Most were older than 65 years, insured, white, and equipped with some college education. Many were enrolled in hospice, though more in Oregon (87.8 percent) than in Washington (64.2 percent), possibly due to the fact that a greater number in Oregon were insured.

While cancer was the most prevalent underlying illness for those seeking MAID, patients most commonly took matters into their own hands due to loss of autonomy (87.4 percent), impaired quality of life/inability to engage in enjoyable activities (86.1 percent), and loss of dignity (68.6 percent). This stood at odds with the commonly expected reasons of inadequate pain control or cost of treatment. While prescribers were present less than 10 percent of time during ingestion, complications were rarely reported.

Charles Blanke, an oncologist in Oregon who has been providing medical aid in dying since 1998 and now has his own end-of-life clinic, said that while early on he didn't think to ask patients if they wanted him present, he now always does, and that most of them welcome the option. "Patients are surprised when I offer," Blanke said. "I don't think they would ever think that it's something that doctors would be willing to do." Blanke said it protects them from investigation if they're not enrolled in hospice; provides an opportunity to address any discomfort, pain, or nausea that might emerge; allows him to explain any common, death-related developments to family members; and relieves family members of the mental and emotional strain of preparing the medication. "Sometimes it's just me and the patient, particularly if they're staying in a nursing home," Blanke said. "Sometimes their family's around and they just quietly sit with each other. Sometimes there are heartfelt speeches. I've had them whip out guitars and ukuleles and play music. I've had some of them sort of throw a little party. It really varies, and it's always just a deeply moving experience."

The situations that Blanke finds most difficult or frustrating are those where the patient seeking medical aid in dying ultimately decides against it because family members are adamantly opposed, or is actually unable to do so because they reach a point where they can no longer ingest the medication on their own. One terrible death involved a young man with several cancer-related fistulas that had connected his large and small bowels, and who was constantly vomiting feces. "He was staring in bed, vomiting stool, staring at his ceiling," said Blanke, who was distressed by not being able to help. "He couldn't interact with his family. He couldn't watch TV. Couldn't read a book. Of course he couldn't eat or drink. And there was nothing we could do to either make him more comfortable or make his time higher quality." Another challenging situation revolved around a patient who was homeless—he had nowhere private to take the medication, so he eventually chose a motel room; while Blanke encouraged him to tell the management ahead of time, he couldn't ensure that would happen. Meanwhile, Blanke said the single most emotionally difficult situation was when he had a young woman's parents and child attend her death. "Having her be young enough to have both children and parents there was hard, even though it's clearly what she wanted," he said.

Early on in his oncology practice, Blanke would wait for patients to broach the question of aid in dying; these days, they seek his services at his end-of-life clinic for that specific purpose. First, he discusses their medical situation and background to determine whether or not they qualify under Oregon's law; then, he explains the statute and who's covered; and finally, he discusses how to make a request for death with dignity. Blanke closes by laying out the patients' options—to turn it down; to keep it in mind but not yet begin the process; or to make the first approval request for lethal medication, after which they must wait fifteen days and do so a second time. "Probably 85 percent of those who are eligible make that first request on the spot," he said.

While Blanke finds the legislation largely effective at protecting patients, he takes issue with the fact that people with disabilities, such as Lou Gehrig's disease, don't qualify because they can't self-administer. With one patient, who only had motion in one finger and in her head, Blanke spent four hours figuring out an approach that worked: He placed a nasogastric tube from her nose to her stomach and attached a syringe; she pressed it with the side of her head to administer the medication.

"That's crazy," he said. "There is no question whatsoever that she wanted to end her life. And just because she couldn't swallow or use her hand, she had to go through these shenanigans to satisfy a statute."

Blanke and others who support MAID are typically advocates of hospice and palliative care and see it as one of several options available to patients at the end of life. DeWolf, referring to Shavelson's Book, *A Chosen Death: The Dying Confront Assisted Suicide*, which outlined the impact on five individuals pursuing MAID at a time when it was not legal in the US, said that their deaths could be compared to back-alley abortions. "Those deaths were botched and miserably handled," she said. "Often with a lot of love and care, but because they had to be secretive, they were what we call 'in darkened bedrooms.'" While death is always sad, she said, her goal is to provide decent, attentive care to patients at the end of life, no matter how they choose to die. Her personal ritual after a patient has died from MAID involves leaving the room to give the family members time to grieve, going into the kitchen to wash her hands, and allowing the tears to come. "I'll walk with people through whatever process they feel they need," she said. "Most of my patients who end up taking medical aid in dying do so because they've just had it—they don't want to keep on going."

"A Step I Can't Go with You"

While clinicians who provide or assist in medical aid in dying can face barriers to providing the care they desire, those who are morally opposed must grapple with ethical quandaries related to their chosen profession, as well as difficult questions around best practices in states where it's legal. Whereas advocates prefer the term "medical aid in dying" (because "suicide" is stigmatizing, and patients who take advantage of the option are already dying), opponents feel that "physician-assisted suicide" (PAS) is the more accurate term. "I just think it's the most straightforward description of what's actually happening," said Daniel Sulmasy, a practicing physician and director of the Kennedy Institute of Ethics at Georgetown University. "A term like medical aid in dying is extremely broad. That includes, for instance, holding some-one's hand; talking to them; telling them that you love them as they are dying a natural death."

Sulmasy said he's never considered MAID/PAS an option. "I have never even thought of it as something conceivable for a physician throughout my now fairly long career," he said. "I think that the trust that's necessary to create a space in which patients are capable of divulg-ing to us their deepest and darkest secrets, and making their bodies naked and presenting them to us in ways that ordinary people don't typ-ically have the experience of, [requires] certain boundaries that have to be absolute. And for me, those are: I will not divulge what you tell me in secret. I will not have sex with you. And I will not kill you." Sulmasy considers the practice bad medicine, in that he believes it shouldn't be necessary if clinicians are doing their job well; bad ethics, because each individual's life has value; and bad public policy, because it doesn't allow for participation from individuals with disabilities and creates a slippery slope where family members or other third parties could eventually begin to choose aid in dying on behalf of their loved ones, or physician-administered euthanasia could become legal.

When patients bring up assistance in dying, Sulmasy said, he engages them in conversation to find out why they are seeking it or what they might be afraid of. He also assures them that palliative care and hospice can address pain and other symptoms. "Most people will, in those kinds of generic conversations, be very satisfied and sometimes surprised to hear how much can actually be done for them," Sulmasy said. In one situation in New York (where MAID/PAS is not legal), the brother of a dying man had wanted the patient to receive assistance in dying. When Sulmasy's team asked why, they learned that it was because the HMO was going to send the patient to a hospice facility in the Bronx, while the brother, who was blind and had difficulty using public transporta-tion, lived in Staten Island. As a result, the hospital arranged to take a lower rate of payment from the HMO to keep the patient in the hos-pital. "If the patient just says, this is what I want, and we think, well, we have to respect their autonomy and I'll do it, and we've never probed the reasons, then I think we're making significant mistakes," said Sulmasy, who was gratified to find an amenable solution. If after discussion a patient continues to insist on assistance in dying, Sulmasy would say, "It's a step I can't go with you . . . but there are resources for you to seek out, and I'm sure you know what they are." He would also express his desire to remain their doctor and to help them live the best quality of life for as long as they have. "I think there is a distinction to be made between killing and allowing a patient to die," said Sulmasy, who is fully supportive of discontinuing treatments such as chemotherapy and life support that are no longer serving the patient.

Ronald Pies, professor emeritus of psychiatry and lecturer on bioethics at SUNY Upstate Medical University in New York, said that he believes that MAID/PAS is not compatible with the medical tradition going back to the time of Hippocrates that forbade physicians from killing patients or helping patients to kill themselves. (Advocates, including Blanke, say the Hippocratic argument doesn't hold weight because it sidesteps other practices, like abortion, that were similarly forbidden at that time, while providing a dignified death is not harming the patient.) While Pies has never been asked about MAID/PAS by a patient, he said that if he were, "I would, instead, explore the patient's reasons for requesting PAS; assess the presence of any treatable psychiatric conditions, such as depression; explore issues of concern to the patient, such as loss of autonomy, loss of dignity, etc.; and provide supportive counseling for those issues." He added that he would ensure the patient received advanced palliative care; and if a mentally competent patient remained intent on ending his or her life, would explore the pros and cons of voluntary stopping of eating and drinking (VSED), in which a patient stops ingesting foods and liquids. "I believe that this kind of response is fully compatible with Hippocratic medical practice, which effectively prohibits physician-assisted suicide," Pies said.

Ira Byock, the founder and chief medical officer of the Institute for Human Caring at Providence St. Joseph Health in Gardena, California, who has a modest stance and compassionate manner, said that he thinks physician-assisted suicide is the wrong subject to be debating. "We should be debating why people don't have universal access to healthcare in general, why people are made to feel badly because they're going through their family's savings in the context of being seriously ill," he said, pointing out that Canada has managed to implement a much more humane approach by providing free healthcare to all its citizens. Byock is concerned by the fact that many terminally ill patients are choosing to end their lives not because of undue pain or suffering, but because they don't want to be a burden to their families or feel undignified. "My worries about the slippery slope are all coming true," he said. "All of the safeguards, all of the waiting periods, psychiatric evaluations, requirements that somebody has to take the medication themselves, requirements that it can't be used with somebody with dementia—every single one of those things has now been recast as a barrier to the right to die."

Like other opponents, Byock takes issue with what he sees as the implication that an unproductive member of society has no real value, purpose, or role to play. "Like it or not, my friends on the other side of this debate are offering a very parsimonious, very parched model of human caring and social support," Byock said, adding that he would like to see well-being at the end of life become the next big thing in American culture. "The fact that we can continue to be well or can sometimes for the first time achieve a sense of well-being during times of decline is something that I've seen quite a bit, but I think the general culture is clueless about it," he said.

Mark O'Rourke, an integrative oncologist in South Carolina who's also certified in hospice and palliative care, has also found that patients can find an unexpected sense of well-being at the end of life and believes that it can be elicited by clinicians who don't join with dying patients' assessment that their life is no longer worth living. "Oftentimes we're just accompanying them on the journey, and helping control their symptoms, but letting them know that they are important to us. And that their life has meaning and we'll take care of them for the time they have," said O'Rourke, choosing his words carefully. "When you're able to connect with people like that, that is a huge relief for people. And it dramatically reduces the suffering." O'Rourke added that while there's a widespread desire not to be a burden and to remain in control of our lives, human beings are, inevitably, dependent on one another. "As children we're born and somebody has to change our diapers and feed us and clothe us and help us, and as frail old people, at some point we lose control of our bowels and somebody has to change our diapers and feed us and take care of us," he said. "So the human condition is not autonomy, but actually interdependence with other people."

In addition to seeing patients from urban and suburban areas, O'Rourke, who practices in the northern part of the state close to foothills in the Piedmont region, sees patients from very rural areas who are quite humble—not only in terms of wealth and assets, but also in terms of support. Not uncommonly, O'Rourke finds himself caring for patients who have no close human relationships, are largely isolated, and have led difficult lives—and he's often impressed by the close relationships they develop with their healthcare team. "They say, 'You know, I've never been treated this well in my whole life. I've never had people care about me or take an interest in me,'" O'Rourke said. While MAID/PAS is not legal in North Carolina or South Carolina, the two states where O'Rourke has practiced for forty years, he will occasionally have patients ask probing questions around the issue. "It's certainly an important thing to respond to," he said of inquiries into MAID/PAS. "There's a world of different things that people worry about [related to dying]—to sort of figure out what they are and address them, and tell patients how we can help them with that."

Chelsia Harris, executive director and associate professor at the School of Nursing at Lipscomb University, a Christian liberal arts institution in Nashville, Tennessee, said that she struggled with the concept of aid in dying when exposed to it as a doctoral student in Ohio—partly because it conflicted with her religious beliefs. "Ethically, there were huge dilemmas there," said Harris, who's spent two decades as a nurse, several years as a nurse practitioner, and over a decade as an educator. "To my background and worldview, it's playing God." In her time as a nurse, Harris witnessed situations in which people given a terminal diagnosis had been healed; perhaps the most dramatic was during her doctoral education, when she was working full-time as a nurse educator and a colleague with metastasized small cell lung cancer came in to speak to her class about palliative care from a patient's perspective. The students prayed for him. Two months later, the colleague—who had sold his home and liquidated his assets to make sure his wife and children were cared for after his death—called to say the cancer was gone; his doctor had no explanation. "I just kept thinking, my goodness, physician-assisted suicide—what if it goes wrong?" Harris said. In addition to unexpected recoveries, she was concerned about those who might suffer complications, or the potential for another person to get ahold of the lethal medication. In 2014, Harris published an article on the issue in the journal *Nursing*, "Physician-Assisted Suicide: A Nurse's Perspective," which pointed out some of these concerns and encouraged nurses to take the time to ascertain their own feelings around MAID/PAS so as to know if they could discuss it in an objective manner or whether they should step aside and allow somebody else to do so.

Over the course of her career, Harris has worked with multiple patients who've expressed the desire to die—including her own father. Once a strong, nearly six-foot-five-inch business owner, her father suffered from kidney failure and diabetes—and once he'd started to go blind, had lost the ability to drive, and found that his independence became impaired "he was finished," Harris said. After spending five days in the hospital due to some foot ulcerations that had gone septic, he went home against medical advice, and "basically told me he was not going back to the hospital. That he was going to sit right there, and he was going to die." Harris asked herself what she would do if she were his nurse and not his daughter. "I would not argue with him," she said. "I would trust what he desires and what he believes is happening." So Harris obeyed her father's wishes—after making sure his neighbors would check him, she left him, as he'd instructed, to his final bowl of ice cream. While her father's decision to decline further treatment killed him within a few hours, Harris saw that as very different from obtaining lethal medication to die—something that would have haunted her. "I just feel like that's a really hard place to put people in, both the provider as well as the family and even the patient," Harris said. "There's just too much potential there for error."

"A Big Decision"

Much of the struggle that clinicians encounter when navigating MAID is that the issue is fraught with moral distress—which can be highly corrosive, as it involves acting against one's own moral compass. Whether it's caused by being unable to prescribe MAID, failing to be present at the bedside, or feeling patients have been undervalued, doctors, nurses, chaplains, and other healthcare workers often find their moral and ethical boundaries tested and their very integrity at stake.

For Catherine Sonquist, who trained at the height of the AIDS epidemic in the San Francisco in the mid-1980s, encountering patients who were suffering greatly and begging for assistance in dying, but being unable to provide it, was tremendously distressing. "We couldn't treat all suffering," Sonquist said. "And there was a medical practice that would be right within our oath to help suffering that would be providing this kind of care, but it was not legal." Later, when Sonquist's own mother was dying and would have partaken in aid in dying were it legal, she asked Sonquist to participate if it ever became possible. Sonquist assisted in drafting the California law, and was among the first to legally prescribe aid in dying in the state. "The idea that we could hasten a death did not feel—has never felt—unethical to me," she said. "This person is going to die anyway. The question is: Are they going to die after suffering or not?"

Those providing or otherwise participating in aid in dying can also experience some moral distress. Oregon's 1999 report on the first year of "Death with Dignity" found that some of the fourteen prescribing physicians shared comments such as "this was really hard on me," and "this had a tremendous emotional impact," while a series of interviews with physicians who had received requests for MAID in Oregon found that they experienced apprehension, discomfort, and emotional intensity.

Chaplains who accompany patients through aid in dying, meanwhile, must find ways to reconcile the practice with their religious or spiritual beliefs. A retired Catholic hospice chaplain who consults with a Honolulu-based hospice on aid in dying under Hawaii's Our Care, Our Choice Act, and who asked not to be identified due to the religious controversy surrounding the issue, said that while he sees aid in dying as an extension of hospice work, he had a strange reaction the first time a patient ingested the medication. The chaplain was at home—having been barred from being at the bedside, along with the other clinicians—but was aware of the time of ingestion, and was waiting for the head nurse to call and let him know that the patient had died. "I didn't know what was happening to me," he said. "I thought I might be having a stroke. I was just really out of it, you know?" After the nurse called, the nausea and disorientation he had been experiencing dissipated—and the chaplain realized he had been distressed. He'd read about the concept of moral distress, or a moral wound, and felt that while he couldn't pinpoint it exactly, "there was something of that in there." While he hasn't experienced anything like that since—and has since been permitted to stay present at the bedside, as he and the other clinicians had protested—the chaplain said that part of what drives him to participate is his desire to better understand the issue. It's hard for him to watch patients ingest the medication, but is also important to him not to abandon patients when they need him most—though those seeking aid in dying, he said, typically have less need of chaplaincy services because they're coming into hospice with their mind already set on what they want. "I want people to have safe opportunities, dignified opportunities, to end their lives," he said. "I hold no judgment for them."

The stance of many medical societies on the issues is somewhat opaque. A 2020 analysis of 150 secular medical and surgical societies in the US found that only 8 percent had position statements on MAID/PAS—with 11 advocating, 5 opposing, and 4 taking a stance of studied neutrality. Notably, the World Medical Association (WMA) and the American Medical Association (AMA) have voiced strong opposition to MAID/PAS, with the WMA stating that "no physician should be forced to participate in euthanasia or assisted suicide, nor should any physician be obliged to make referral decisions to this end." Nevertheless, the AMA's code of ethics states that "Supporters and opponents share a fundamental commitment to values of care, compassion, respect, and dignity; they diverge in drawing different moral conclusions from those underlying values in equally good faith." In 2019, the American Nurses Association (ANA) revised its position to reflect the growing legality of aid in dying and advised nurses to take an objective stance when discussing the option with patients.

Felicia Stokes, a senior policy advisor for the ANA's Center for Ethics and Human Rights, said that in preparation for the five-year update on its position, the ANA took several member surveys. "Nurses would say, 'Well, what does it mean to participate? We need to understand ethically what that means,'" Stokes said. In a separate study that the ANA conducted with UCSF, Stokes said preliminary data showed that many nurses had no idea that medical aid in dying existed, even in states where it's legal. "There's certainly an education gap," she said, pointing out that MAID education for nurses is often not perceived as necessary because nurses don't write the prescriptions—but they're often the ones at the bedside when the patients bring it up. Stokes believes that state laws for MAID should fund education for both physicians and nurses. "They're really walking into these situations blindly," she said of nurses. "It is quite concerning and quite alarming."

Eventually, as in other countries such as Canada, nurse practitioners may even be able to write prescriptions for MAID; Hawaii is considering legislation allowing them to do so. In a 2017 paper exploring such a possibility for *The Journal for Nurse Practitioners*, Stokes cited studies that show how 1 to 18 percent of nurses directly hastened a patient's death through intentionally injecting, or illegally providing or prescribing drugs. Stokes said that this is likely due to the empathy that nurses feel for their patients, and that she's personally had patients grab her arm, saying "Please help me. I don't want to continue to live like this." Such situations can cause significant moral distress—particularly when they're happening repeatedly, she said. "It's a huge, huge problem in nursing, and one that causes nurses to leave the profession—not being able to really reckon with watching someone die and feeling helpless and feeling like you can't do enough, or you haven't done enough, to help alleviate that person's suffering."

Stokes said that some institutions have begun having moral distress rounds—where a nurse can page a clinical ethicist or similar specialist to come guide the nurses in thinking through and processing the situation, as well as provide resilience strategies—and that these are highly effective. "You're teaching nurses about ethics and values, but you're also teaching them about resilience and how to strengthen their resilience through individual methods of stepping away," she said. This is essential because nurses experience quick patient turnover—even after a death—and are rarely given time to engage in prayer, mindfulness, a walk, or some other useful activity, she said.

Recently, Stokes also polled nurses to see if *slow codes* (i.e., situations in which clinicians decide to not aggressively resuscitate a terminally ill patient by moving slower than they would during a usual code) were still happening. They were—largely, she found, due to moral distress. "They did it out of a place of goodness for their patients, so they wouldn't cause harm to their patients," she said. Slow codes are highly controversial, as are some other methods of failing to prolong life, such as voluntary stopping eating and drinking (VSED) and even palliative sedation. Many patients naturally stop eating and drinking at the end of life, and most clinicians agree that it's important not to force food and water at this time. Yet some—including Sulmasy, the ethicist at Georgetown University—stand in strong opposition to choosing VSED well in advance of death or administering sedation with the explicit purpose of making patients unconscious in order to hasten death. "I think it's just a slow form of physician-assisted suicide," he said.

Meanwhile, advocates such as Dena Davis, the presidential endowed chair in health and professor of bioethics at Lehigh University in Pennsylvania, believes right-to-die measures are more stringent than they should be, and that the moral distress experienced by healthcare workers could actually harm patients who are seeking to stop aggressive end-of-life measures. Davis, whose mother suffered from dementia for years before she died, fears that if she became demented, she would not only be unable to access MAID—as one has to be both of sound mind and within six months of death—but that even her advance directive, which might refuse treatments such as antibiotics for pneumonia, could be dishonored by nursing home staff experiencing moral distress around the fact that it was written when she was competent. As a result, Davis believes that the best option for those diagnosed with Alzheimer's who place strong value on avoiding the years between diagnosis and death is to preemptively end their own lives, whether or not it's legal. "I know it's kind of a radical belief," Davis said. "It isn't to me."

While right-to-die advocates can see moral distress as a barrier to care, opponents often cite moral distress as indicative of the fact that clinicians should not be participating in MAID/PAS. Still others see it as a natural outgrowth of walking a challenging edge. "I think it's a stretching experience to work in this zone," Quill said. "If you didn't have any angst as you're going through this, I'd think there's something wrong with you." He said that the need to navigate moral distress, and determine the best outcome for patients, is part of the reason he believes so strongly in an open process around MAID, and that if he was experiencing severe moral distress over prescribing lethal medication, he wouldn't do it. In general, though, he sees it as "the same moral distress when I'm taking somebody off of life support, which we all agree is permissible. But, you know, people die as a result of this decision. So it's a big decision."

12

It Takes a Village

What do we live for, if it is not to make life less difficult for
each other?

—GEORGE ELIOT

The first time Karren Ganschinietz—who spent more than thirty years
as a CNA in assisted living, home health, and private duty—entered a
resident's room at a skilled nursing facility, she had a big smile on her
face, ready to offer him a warm washcloth and breakfast. To her shock,
the 102-year-old man called her a "white cracker," and threw his urinal
at her, drenching her. Ganschinietz, who has wavy, red-brown hair and a
kindly crease to her eyes, was furious. She closed her eyes and clenched
her fists. "I felt, 'how could this person do this?'" she said. "Does he not
know that I'm here to help him?" Yet Ganschinietz's anger was directed
not at the resident—a large man named Jim, who'd lost his left leg as a
youth under unclear circumstances—but at the nurse who'd failed to
warn her. "I didn't take it personally," said Ganschinietz, who returned to
the resident's room—where he continued to hurl his urine at her for the
next six months, until he learned to trust her. "I knew in his generation

there were a lot of difficulties, and I just learned to accept it." Eventually, the two of them established a bond—Jim would request Ganschinietz, and they would joke around. "He would say, 'Now you know I have my urinal,'" she said. "And I'd say, 'Yep. And you know I have an extra uniform in my locker.' And we'd just chuckle."

Ganschinietz worked with Jim for about two years before transferring to a new position. When she told him she had some bad news, he asked her if she'd been fired, or knocked up. She told him no, she was leaving—and he started to cry. "He kissed me on the forehead and said, 'Don't forget about me,'" Ganschinietz said. She went back to see Jim several times. On her first visit, she brought him red tulips; Jim had always wanted his windows open, so that he could see the tulips blooming outside. About six months later, he died. "I was kind of relieved that he had passed because his suffering was gone, but yet it was like losing a friend," Ganschinietz said. "Even though I was his caregiver, we had that friendship bond."

While doctors and nurses are the most publicly acknowledged healthcare workers, there are numerous others in the trenches who receive much less consideration, recognition—and pay. Home health aides and CNAs, including Ganschinietz, become close to residents through intimate, daily encounters, while often enduring name-calling and other forms of abuse. Meanwhile, the grief and trauma experienced by orderlies, medical interpreters, medical assistants, environmental service workers, and others in less recognized positions can be highly disenfranchised as they are often overlooked when it comes to formal mechanisms for processing emotions, such as huddles or debriefings. Such auxiliary staff also often receive less compensation and limited benefits, stressors that only heighten their burden.

Volunteers and other nonclinical staff, meanwhile, provide widespread assistance, offering patients pet therapy, art therapy, music, and massage. These varied offerings—many of which are unpaid—afford immense relief to clinicians by enhancing patients' moods, improving their willingness to connect with providers, and eliciting a sense of joy, engagement, or calm among patients and staff alike. One additional—and not insignificant—challenge posed by the COVID-19 pandemic was that many hospitals, hospices, nursing homes, and other facilities had to temporarily halt their volunteer programs, reducing the environment to one that was even more grim. "Organizations cannot possibly put a value on a volunteer," said Karla Bachl, director of volunteer services for Lehigh Valley Health Network in Pennsylvania. "We're helping the humanistic part of healthcare to the fullest. It's not a pill, it's not a treatment, it's not a procedure—it's an emotion."

Part of what healthcare settings can do to buttress their workers includes recognizing, including, and financially supporting less visible staff; embracing the cooperation provided by volunteers; and enlisting more nonclinical support to perform duties such as stocking supplies, acting as scribes, or simply sitting with patients. Such assistance can prove particularly poignant when patients are dying, allowing clinicians to know that someone's at the bedside when a patient has no family present, or that newly bereaved family members have additional help. Yet organizations must also recognize that all volunteers and staff are affected by the grief and trauma witnessed in the healthcare setting and take measures to provide necessary emotional, mental, and spiritual support.

"Give Us the Same Treatment"

Beatriz Juarez had spent more than five years as a Spanish language medical interpreter at a Level 1 trauma center in New Mexico when something snapped. Working nights and weekends, she'd seen terrible things—people who'd been shot, car accidents, stillborn babies. Once, she'd interpreted for the grandparents of a little girl who'd been shot in a road rage incident; the grandfather blamed himself for not picking her up from school as he usually did. Often, Juarez would have to deliver bad news to family members—such as the parents of a young man, who'd been killed while intoxicated and drag racing on Father's Day. Unlike other healthcare staff, who could avoid specialties such as pediatrics that they found too challenging, Juarez experienced it all. "We as interpreters don't have the luxury of saying, 'I can't do this type of encounter,'"

Juarez said. Meanwhile, interpreters were often sent into dramatic situations with little-to-no preparation. "I would just go in and on the spot would have to take that all in," she said, her dark, almond-shaped eyes widening. "And then as soon as I would walk out of their room, I would have another call waiting."

Still, Juarez handled it fairly well until one Saturday night in July 2018, when a bus, which had been traveling from Colorado to Ciudad Juárez, Mexico, collided with a semi; some forty injured people, largely Spanish-speaking, ended up at her hospital. "A lady arrived without an arm," Juarez said. "Another lady, her legs were almost completely torn apart. And I got overwhelmed." As the only interpreter on duty, Juarez felt unable to provide appropriate care—rather than staying with one patient until they went to the ICU or the operating room, the way she usually did, she was jumping from person to person, translating rapid-fire questions about allergies and past surgeries. One man begged her to locate his wife, who had also been on the bus, and she promised to do so—then promptly forgot, as she had to attend to a multitude of other patients. The one woman that Juarez thought was doing well turned out to have a spinal injury. "I felt like I didn't do enough," said Juarez, who had called some colleagues to come in and help. "That was part of the guilt."

Juarez went home at 8 a.m. the next morning and couldn't sleep. Three days later she still wasn't sleeping, so she went to the employee urgent care; they sent her to the psychiatric ER, where they gave her hydroxyzine for sleep and asked her to follow up with a psychologist, whom Juarez began seeing weekly. She started having panic attacks, regular nightmares, and visual hallucinations—shortly after the incident, Juarez took a previously planned vacation with her family to Los Cabos, Mexico, where she hallucinated alligators swimming next to her in the ocean. She often felt short of breath, and began having twitches in her eyebrow, lip, and legs. She went to see a hypnotherapist, which helped, but she was still seeing traumas at work and taking medications for anxiety and depression. About a year after the bus incident, she began working days, which typically had fewer traumatic incidents. Then in October 2020, she switched to a job at a different hospital: a supervisory role with some remote interpreting. Still, when Juarez—who'd been diagnosed with chronic PTSD six months after the bus incident—tried to stop her medications, the symptoms returned. "I don't know if it was already accumulating in my system, and that was, like they said, the last drop that filled my glass," she said. "Or if that was the only incident that I didn't know how to deal with and it made me go into this internal chaos." Juarez said that while her hospital's emergency department had held a debriefing following the bus incident—as well as for some earlier, exceptionally traumatic situations she'd worked—as a medical interpreter, she hadn't been included. Meanwhile, she rarely saw her colleagues except for a short exchange when her shift was ending. "We are not really considered part of a group because we're everywhere," she said. "I would have no one to debrief." Juarez added that following her experience, the hospital had begun initiating changes to include medical interpreters in debriefings.

Xiomara Armas, who has been working at Children's Healthcare of Atlanta for more than fifteen years, provides both in-person and remote Spanish interpreting services for children and their families. While Armas enjoys working in pediatrics, she said some patients can be hard to move on from, particularly children who succumb to aggressive cancers. One that impacted her deeply was an eight-year-old boy from El Salvador. His family was undocumented and unable to afford the bone marrow transplant he required; the hospital's social workers couldn't find resources to help him. Armas worked with the family for two years up until he died. Afterward, "I just felt that part of me was broken," she said. Armas met with chaplains in the hospital's chapel to discuss her distress around the fact that someone so young, with his whole life ahead of him, had died. "They were a lot of help for me," she said, adding that she appreciated "the time that they take to listen and orient your feelings in a positive way." Armas, who serves as chair for the National Board of Certification for Medical Interpreters, said that to take care of herself she gardens, growing flowers as well as cucumbers, tomatoes, carrots, and other vegetables. She enjoys spending time with her husband and their two dogs, or taking meandering walks along the Chattahoochee River.

Inspired by an ICU physician who found painting the water on his days off to be uplifting, Armas said she'd like to take up painting next. "I love the colors," she said.

While medical interpreters can be exposed to a wide variety of traumas and grief-inducing situations, sometimes with very little emotional support, environmental service (EVS) workers—who clean and disinfect patients' rooms as well as other areas of the hospital—often become attached to patients they see on a regular basis. Carmencita Smith, a diminutive woman with a hearty laugh who's been working in the industry for more than thirty years, said that she used to work closely with cancer patients, and that it was hard for her to witness their suffering—especially when there were no family members present. "Every day I see them, [when] I clean. And every time before they sleep, they'll say, 'I want to see you before I sleep,'" she said. "When the patient dies that you're very close to, it breaks your heart." Smith, who now works at the Swedish Medical Center in Seattle, said that when EVS staff feel recognized—through simple things like an announcement, or a special celebratory event—it makes a big difference in their ability to show up for patients. After work Smith likes to relax, listen to music, and tidy up and decorate her house.

During the COVID-19 pandemic, EVS workers were often the last in line—not only in receiving recognition from the general public, but also more practical support such as PPE. "They don't understand that we pick up the contaminated linen, the garbage that has soiled things," said Angel Sherburne, also an EVS worker at the Swedish Medical Center. Toward the beginning of the pandemic, she said, EVS staff had to push to get testing and proper PPE, including N-95 masks. Meanwhile, some EVS workers didn't want to clean rooms that had housed patients infected with the virus, meaning Sherburne—a highly experienced worker who'd previously been a supervisor in the Philippines—had to clean more of them. At the end of 2020, Sherburne contracted the virus, coming down with chills, a fever, and a cough; after she recovered, she became fully vaccinated. "They need to give us the same treatment as the other healthcare workers," Sherburne said, adding that she'd like to see EVS and other workers at the hospital receive hazard pay.

In addition to better benefits and opportunities to process grief and loss, many overlooked healthcare workers say that simple recognition and an ability to be heard can make a significant difference in preventing burnout. Cat Clohessy, a CNA on an oncology unit in Northern California, said that her hospital has weekly check-ins during which staff talk about using their skills, if they're feeling valued, things that they enjoy doing, and things that they've found challenging. Regular check-ins "really facilitate that conversation," she said. "It's also a really good tool for mentors to be able to give you credit where credit is due." Clohessy added that the hospital also has something called "Wildcards," which staff can write for one another when someone does something that stands out, like helping out a colleague or providing exceptional patient care. "It's definitely nice, especially when sometimes you're just running around and you've had a crazy day, to have your coworkers just be like, 'Hey, I see you,'" she said.

Whether recognition and support come from supervisors, peers, or patients, they're always valued and are what get many healthcare workers through their most trying moments. Ganschinietz, the long-time CNA, said that CNAs would often support each other when residents died; conventional wisdom was that "they travel in threes," meaning that three residents typically died per month. On her days off, Ganschinietz would sometimes get a text message asking if she preferred to receive bad news by text or by telephone. When a resident died that a CNA had been particularly close to, the others would cover for that staff member so that they could "take a little bit of time to go talk to the family members or just to collect themselves," she said. Some managers were more supportive of this practice than others, Ganschinietz said, emphasizing that CNAs should be given more time to grieve and a longer lag time before a new resident is placed in the room. "If a CNA is dealing pretty poorly with the loss of a resident, they need to allow that person to take one or two days off," she said. "They need to take into consideration that this person is part of our family, part of our lives." Like CNAs, EVS workers, medical interpreters, orderlies, and other less-recognized staff also have unique patient relationships resulting in grief and trauma—and often, less formal time to process.

"Just So Grateful"

One key layer of support for both patients and clinicians comes in the form of volunteers and nonclinical staff. Evidence shows that volunteers in hospitals save organizations money while contributing to an improvement in patient satisfaction scores. Yet they also assist doctors, nurses, and other healthcare workers by calming distraught children, engaging patients who are withdrawn, or sitting with the dying. Many times, healthcare staff are relieved to have someone who can stock supplies, bring a patient a glass of water, or read to sick children. Meanwhile, clinicians can also benefit directly from exposure to calming activities such as music, art, massage, and pet therapy.

Shelly Niebuhr, a kindly woman with a soft-spoken, thoughtful manner, spent two decades providing music for patients in hospitals, rehabilitation centers, skilled nursing facilities, memory care facilities, and other healthcare settings in Dallas—at least half that time as a certified music practitioner. She started in acute care settings through an arts program in 2001 and moved on to work with patients with all kinds of conditions—some were critically ill or actively dying; others had brain injuries or were homebound with rheumatoid arthritis. Niebuhr was impressed to see the impact that playing guitar and singing had on disgruntled patients. "Suddenly they would do their physical therapy," she said. "With memory care, it was huge—where they don't know their own name, but suddenly they're singing all these songs." She would sometimes incorporate an Irish flute and, for large groups, the mandolin, harmonica, and various forms of percussion.

Niebuhr said the music was prescriptive, and it would vary—it would be different for an acutely ill patient, for example, than for one who was dying. For someone with dementia, she'd play familiar music; for someone who was critically ill, she'd try to follow their heartbeat, using major keys and moving from song to song without long pauses. "If the person is dying, depending on what stage they're in, then you play music that's typically unmetered or without a countable beat," she said. "Because if you go in to a dying person and you just start playing something, that can really agitate them, it can make their process much worse." Niebuhr would sometimes improvise and match their breathing. "You can just really see them calming down, getting peaceful, smiling," she said. "I always left feeling humbled in the very best sense."

Clinicians were positively impacted by the music she played as well. Many told Niebuhr that it had helped to reduce their anxiety, allowing them to slow down, take a deep breath, and better connect with their patients. Other times, the music enabled them to see patients in a different, more humanizing, way. Sometimes Niebuhr would be working with a patient with a brain injury, and the doctor would get excited by the patient's response—they would start making eye contact or try to sing along.

Other patients proved much more difficult; occasionally, they even tried to physically attack her. "You're dealing with people when they're at their worst," Niebuhr said. "They're in pain, they're frightened. They may be angry with you; they may be completely withdrawn." One young woman, who'd become a quadriplegic and blind following a car accident, would cry incessantly; Niebuhr worked with her individually to find music that soothed her. "She still haunts me," Niebuhr said. Sometimes, Niebuhr encountered patients the music couldn't reach—such as the young man who'd been electrocuted by a power line and was kept in an enclosure bed with mesh walls because he was so crazed. "You don't forget that kind of suffering when you see it," said Niebuhr, who prayed for her patients and relied on meditation to keep her grounded. "You can't." Niebuhr found that the work changed the way she lived: She now experiences some anxiety when driving, and while she used to love to ride horses, she "would never dream of getting on a horse again." Volunteers and staff, such as Niebuhr, not only face difficult clinical situations, but are also impacted in long-term, life-changing ways.

Another calming modality utilized in healthcare settings is massage. Gayle MacDonald, who has short, gray hair and a forthright style, was leading a massage class in Oregon in the early 1990s when a Portland hospital called and asked her students to serve as volunteers for its oncology patients. Shortly after, they established an ongoing program; eventually, it received funding. The patients MacDonald massaged enjoyed it so much that they often asked her to come live with them or told her that she had the hands of an angel. Once, a nurse asked MacDonald to accompany a mother whose twenty-one-year-old was about to be put on a ventilator in the ICU. "I didn't exactly know how to do that, but I just stood behind her with my hands on her shoulders and just did a little light kind of compression and release," MacDonald said. "She was just so grateful to have that kind of presence as she watched her son be intubated." Contrary to expectations, the woman's son survived, and MacDonald stayed in touch with his mother for years afterward. "An experience like that, it just glues you together," she said.

While massage therapy was once considered a core nursing skill, growing technological and documentation demands caused it to fall by the wayside in the mid-twentieth century. But recently, more institutions have been recognizing its value in keeping patients and their caregivers connected, while improving patients' pain management and stress levels, and promoting healing, relaxation, and sleep. Meanwhile, healthcare staff benefit from the presence of massage therapists as well. "The staff will say, 'Okay, you be sure you tell Mrs. Smith that I was the one that sent you in there' so that the nurse gets the brownie points," MacDonald said. Occasionally, nurses benefit more directly: when waiting for patients to return from a scan, MacDonald would sometimes give them a quick massage, as well. "What they always asked for was their shoulders," MacDonald said. "And really, sometimes two minutes is all it takes to just get the nurse to go: *Ahh*," she breathed, flopping her own shoulders back and down.

Clinicians are also strongly affected by the presence of trained animals, which bring joy and calm to patients and staff alike. Diane Pekarek, who coordinates the Pet Pals program for fifteen University Hospitals throughout northeast Ohio, said that when their 150 dogs, single cat, and miniature horse were barred from entering the facilities during the COVID-19 pandemic, she would bring several of the dogs and the cat up to the front windows so that hospital staff could have contactless visits. "That's how much staff loved the animals," she said. "And that's how dedicated the volunteers were. And then the dogs would have little signs that their handler made, saying 'We Ruff You' and 'UH Nurses are the best.'" Meanwhile, Pekarek organized virtual visits over iPads for the patients and started a cart of thirteen multicolored GloFish that could be wheeled from room to room. "Staff look forward to that, and they like to just sit and watch," Pekarek said. "It's like watching a campfire with all the colors. You just lose yourself for a couple of minutes."

When the dogs began returning to the lobbies about a year into the pandemic, staff were overjoyed; many cried. The program had everything from a 3-pound Pomeranian to a 175-pound Great Dane, and Pekarek—when evaluating whether or not they were ready to return—addressed the dogs in the same manner the staffers would. "I do a really high-pitched: 'Oh my God,'" she said, her voice transforming into a Valley Girl shriek. "I do that high pitch to get them ready for it." In addition to the volunteer therapy dogs, one hospital had two facility dogs—Melena and Starbucks—who were allowed to remain during the pandemic; Pekarek would take them around to visit with the staff. "You'll have doctors walking down the hallway who will just grab a dog and lean down and cry into them for a few seconds," she said. "The dogs, the animals, allow us to release our emotions and be real."

In addition to directly supporting staff, the therapy animals also provide immense assistance in helping clinicians connect with their patients—especially children. "We've had children that don't want to get out of bed, that don't want to talk," Pekarek said. "They don't want to eat. They've just shut down." One little boy, Jackson, who had to visit the hospital weekly for an excruciating procedure, was much more willing knowing Melena would be there. A child who needed physical therapy didn't want to get up and walk because it was painful but was convinced when told he could walk the miniature horse, Willie Nelson—a patient, stoic animal with meticulously groomed black fur—down the hallway. Once, the cat, a fluffy silver creature named Pearl, who'd been visiting a young girl for months, went to see her just before she died. Even though the girl was unresponsive, she moved her hand to pet Pearl once more before she passed. Patients as well as staff collect and trade baseball-sized cards picturing the animals; new ones are produced every few months. "Staff usually line the nurse's station with them," Pekarek said. "They're like gold around here."

During the COVID-19 pandemic, some individuals came up with creative ways to address the unmet need in healthcare settings that had furloughed both two-legged and four-legged volunteers. Sudan Eubanks, a teenage beauty pageant contestant living in Florida, and her sister, Cairo—Miss Broward County—realized that hospitals had lost their volunteers and didn't see anybody offering virtual programming. The sisters stepped in to create Reading with Royalty, which provided videos of people reading children's books to area hospitals. Initially, most participants were girls in the pageant circuit, but the program quickly expanded to include five hundred volunteers from seven countries. "We've gotten feedback that the different voices, the different ages, the different backgrounds of the readers help the children feel more connected to the outside world," Cairo Eubanks said. Sudan Eubanks added that many have read books in Spanish, which has been great for the Spanish-speaking families in South Florida. "Miss Iowa 2019, she actually sang her book because it was more like a rhyme, and she's a very talented singer," Sudan Eubanks said.

Many healthcare organizations say that volunteer services are, in fact, essential. In neonatal intensive care units (NICUs), volunteers often act as "cuddlers"; holding and soothing premature babies whose parents may be working or otherwise indisposed. Lisa Barnett, a staff nurse in the NICU at Northern Light Health in Eastern Maine, said that their program started many years prior at the impetus of a nurse named Amy Carter; they're known as "Carter's Quiet Care Cuddlers." Some fifteen to twenty volunteers, mostly senior citizens, receive specialized training before participating in the program; one in particular has stepped up to take leadership over the group. Babies who are going through drug withdrawals can be particularly inconsolable, said Barnett, who despite her steady gaze and efficient manner can become overwhelmed. "I can't tell you how many times I've been at the end of my rope," she said. "And if the cuddler walks in, I'm just like: Okay. So happy."

Jay Kerecman, one of the hospital's four neonatologists, said that the cuddlers' presence has likely cut down on the need to provide opiates to babies with extreme withdrawal symptoms, while in general their support is a huge boon to families who can live many hours away. The NICU typically has anywhere from fifteen to nearly thirty babies, some of whom stay for days while others require months of care, he said. Kerecman enjoys living and working in a small community and displays a fatherly manner toward the many people he's cared for as babies—including Barnett's own daughter, who's now in dental school—as well as staff on the transport mission he organizes, which has to overcome challenges such as winter blizzards to bring babies in from very rural areas. Despite the fact that Kerecman has worked in large cities including San Antonio, Texas, and Washington, DC, he said Northern Light Health has the best cuddler program he's seen due to the efficiency of their communication and leadership. Cuddlers "may hold babies, they may feed babies," he said. "I've seen them reading to them, providing some of those things that our nurses can be too busy to do with their assignment load."

While he appreciates the support that volunteers provide to staff, Kerecman said one thing that boosts his own sense of well-being is doing volunteer work himself; in fact, many physicians have identified volunteering in their spare time as a key method to prevent burnout. "I throw myself into that, maybe as a distraction from the issues here," said Kerecman, who teaches guitar to service members with PTSD through a program called Guitars for Vets. "I find that rewarding in of itself, to go and put my energies into something that's completely different from what I do on a daily basis."

No One Dies Alone

While volunteers bring a wide variety of services to the healthcare setting, they can prove particularly crucial to clinicians whose patients are dying—providing an essential presence at the bedside, consolation to bereaved family members, and other support that healthcare staff may not have the time or opportunity to deliver. In the mid-1980s, on a rainy night in Oregon, a nurse named Sandra Clarke was at the bedside of an elderly patient near death when he asked her, in a frail, tremulous voice, to stay with him. Clarke—an earnest woman whose short, white hair ends in dyed ebony points like pencil tips—promised to come back after checking on her six other patients. But by the time she did so, he'd died—alone, with his arm outstretched. "The sense of frustration and anger was overwhelming," Clarke said in a Mayo Clinic video years later. "He had a simple wish that was easily granted, and I couldn't do it." She paused, blinking back tears. "And from that moment on, it became something important to me, to find a way that we could be with patients at the end of life. And I looked around—I mean, you've got kitchen workers, you've got nurses, CNAs, whatever. Couldn't somebody take a moment and be with this person, and give him some comfort at the end?"

Clarke began considering the possibility of creating a volunteer group made up of hospital employees to sit with patients dying alone. In 2001, her idea finally came to fruition as the No One Dies Alone (NODA) program, first implemented at Sacred Heart Medical Center in Eugene. Since then, numerous healthcare organizations around the country have adopted the program, which can include hospital staff as well as outside volunteers who typically sit in three- or four-hour shifts at the bedsides of the dying.

Brian Zenger, codirector of the NODA program at the University of Utah, where he is also a dual MD/PhD student, was drawn to participate because he was interested in learning from the chaplains who ran it—their ability to meet patients seeking spiritual connection, to openly interact with individuals from all faith backgrounds, and to love with detachment. As a volunteer who has sat with ten to fifteen people who are dying, Zenger will often come in and "mess up" a room by unfolding blankets and moving things around, so that if individuals regain consciousness, they'll be able to see that someone's been there. Sometimes, he'll read from materials in one of the purple duffel bags the hospital provides to volunteers, containing a range of religious texts, poetry, and other inspirational items, as well as a journal in which they can note thoughts and reflections. Often, he'll try to match the patient's breathing pattern. "This is deeply personal and we really encourage and rely on our volunteers to be paying attention to physical signs and symptoms," Zenger said, adding that someone who is dying will show signs of agitation when they don't like something, such as squirming, moving away from touch, or disquieted breathing. "No science there, no numbers, no data," he said. "Just a feeling."

Zenger said that the program involves diverse participants—from eighteen-year-olds to seventy-five-year-olds; from students to working professionals and retired people—and has received a great deal of positive feedback from clinicians. "It's one of the most depressing things in the world to get up from a room where a patient's alone," he said. "And that weighs on everybody, no matter who you are in terms of the healthcare team. You could be a nurse, a CNA, a provider, all the way down the janitorial staff." Sometimes, a really distressed provider will call the NODA program and say that a volunteer needs to be there right away. Other times, the service can be solicited through a consult order, or by checking a box when the patient goes on comfort care measures. For clinicians, "it allows you to go on," Zenger said. "You don't get stuck thinking about a patient you left, and it allows you to perform your clinical duties to the best of your ability." The volunteers are supported by gathering together for a dinner every three months at which they engage in some kind of continuing education piece—related to death and dying, or to self-care—before ending with a ritual. Volunteers share thoughts and experiences about the patients they've sat with, such as their surprise at one dying individual's penchant for loud heavy metal music. "It kind of provides that closure and that community support," Zenger said.

Karla Bachl, the director of volunteer services at Lehigh Valley Health Network, said their NODA program has been operating for more than fifteen years, with up to one hundred volunteers, some of whom are hospital staff, at any given time. Bachl said that volunteers take a class on what to expect in the dying process and are given a tote bag with materials, including inspirational readings and prayers, to which they can add personal items such as books or puzzles. Bachl—who left nursing school back in the 1980s in part because the deaths of her cancer patients were too upsetting—said she knows how important such backup can be. "The nurses just love it, and physicians as well," she said. "They do not have the ability to sit with someone for hours and hold their hand while they pass."

Other volunteer organizations focus on family members who've lost a loved one. Missy Thomas, the director of programs at Colorado-based Now I Lay Me Down to Sleep (NILMDTS), which provides complimentary portrait sessions nationally to parents whose babies have died before, during, or shortly after childbirth, said she realized the importance of the service after a close friend lost her full-term baby because he'd been deprived of oxygen for too long during a complicated delivery. The parents hired a photographer to produce images of their family with the baby that they could share. "There was only a handful of family that were able to be [present at the bedside] that quickly," Thomas said. "But the rest of us met him through those photos."

Thomas said that NILMDTS typically works with labor and delivery or NICU nurses, but occasionally also physicians, social workers, chaplains, or child-life specialists who call them to come in. The nonprofit has developed a course for nurses and other healthcare staff, which they can take for continuing education credit, focused on developing their photography skills. "A lot of nurses were taking these photos on their own," Thomas said. "We knew, from a professional photography standpoint, that we can't get them up to a professional photography level of skills, but we also knew that there are a few little tips and tricks, here and there, that can make a huge difference." The program also teaches the research behind remembrance photography—how it helps establish a family identity for parents who may later have to respond to questions like, "Do you have children?" In addition, participants learn tips for communicating with family members (such as using the terms "mom" and "dad," and offering photography early on in the delivery process when appropriate) and for physically handling the baby—something many feel comfortable doing, but that others have less experience with. Even nurses who've been working with newborns for fifteen or twenty years often come away with some new knowledge, Thomas said. "I get a lot of good feedback on that—like 'Oh, I had no idea that you could use a 4×4 gauze pad to prop a baby's chin closed,'" she said.

In addition to her current role, Thomas has worked as a dispatcher and as a photographer for the nonprofit. She's photographed many dozens of families and finds it incredibly rewarding to be able to accompany parents and their babies at such a challenging time. "We know that we can't bring their baby back, we can't change what has happened, but we can give them something with our talents," said Thomas, adding that the photos are edited—not for any genetic abnormalities, but to retouch things like skin peeling and tearing that may have resulted from the birth process. "A lot of the parents are so grateful that they get photos they can actually show to people." Thomas said that while every situation is different, parents are often in shock, or even afraid to hold their baby. Part of what an NILMDTS photography session does is to normalize the relationship so that parents feel more comfortable cradling, talking to, or otherwise devoting attention to the baby. While many are in rough shape, Thomas, who herself has tight brown curls and rosy cheeks, will point out their adorable aspects—such as their toes, or their hair. "We try to pull out the little details," she said. "And we also take photos of those details so that they can remember them later."

One volunteer leader in healthcare, Kate Munger, has taken this gentle treatment typically afforded babies at the beginning of life and applied it to how all individuals are treated at the end. In November of 1990, Munger was asked to take care of a friend who was dying of AIDS. In the morning she did chores, and in the afternoon she was asked to sit at his bedside. "I was terrified because he was unconscious, comatose, but thrashing and agitated," she said. "And so I did what I do when I'm afraid, which is I sing." Munger sang "There's a Moon" by Gail Vail McDermott—and then she repeated it for the next two and a half hours because she saw that it was making him calmer. As he became calmer, so did she. "I felt like I was offering a lullaby," she said. "A very peaceful, comforting lullaby."

Ten year later, Munger started the first Threshold Choir in the Bay Area, which, at the request of caregivers or healthcare staff, visits those who are dying in hospitals, hospices, or in other settings and sings to them a cappella, in harmony. The choirs—typically composed of three to four women at the bedside, and later expanded to include all genders—quickly multiplied, spreading beyond the Bay Area and across the country. Most of their simple, evocative songs were written by the members themselves; often, while sitting with someone who was dying. Other times, dying individuals would ask for songs that were popular when they were in their teens and twenties. When educating healthcare organizations about their offering, Munger, who is now retired, would sit a nurse or a social worker down in a chair and sing to them so that they could experience it on a kinesthetic or spiritual level. "There's something really special that happens when you're sung to," she said, adding that many clinicians would shed a tear or two. "Very often they are at a loss for words, and they don't want to open their eyes. They don't want to come back."

The first time that Raymond Dougherty, director of spiritual care services at Kaiser Permanente in the Marin/Sonoma service area, heard the Threshold Choir, he was attending an annual day of remembrance for all the patients who'd died during the previous year; the names of those patients, along with some of the loved ones that staff had lost, scrolled on a large screen. The Threshold Choir—which defines its music as a healing gift, or a form of prayer, rather than a performance—faced away from the audience, and sang toward those names. "It was just so moving," Dougherty said. "It brought tears to my eyes, seeing the names of some of the patients that I remembered and seeing the care and the beauty that they were bringing to those people." Afterward, Dougherty asked the choir to come see an unresponsive patient he'd recently sat with who was dying in the hospital without friends or family present. "Frankly, I think the music touches into something that's even deeper than maybe some prayers that I could do," Dougherty said. "Because what they're doing is they are taking the words that I would say—the blessings or the affirmations, the good intentions or goodwill that I would be bringing—and they're repeating it over and over again, in three-part harmony: 'Peace be with you'; 'Be not afraid'; 'Go in peace'; 'Know that you are not alone.'"

In addition to patients, Dougherty soon noted that staff, too, found the music incredibly soothing. And in the summer of 2018, he helped conduct a study investigating the impact of the Threshold Choir's singing on nurses and other healthcare workers on a medical-surgical unit. Following the intervention, researchers found that staff noted a statistically significant improvement in centeredness, calmness, peacefulness, and connectedness with patients. "They would take a moment, maybe put down what they're doing," Dougherty said. "Their shoulders would drop, or they'd smile, or take a deep breath and a sigh." Dougherty regularly encouraged staff to integrate such moments of self-care into their workflow, emailing them tips for ways to calm their nervous systems and feel refreshed called "Soul Snacks." One popular "Soul Snack" involved "Shaking and Dancing"—a minute of each, accompanied by music, with a minute of silence in between.

Dougherty said that his colleagues really began appreciating the power of self-care and spiritual care after the hospital shut down for more than three weeks due to the devastating 2017 wildfires. Thousands of people in the Marin-Sonoma area lost their homes. "It was very traumatic for our community," Dougherty said. "There probably wasn't a department where somebody—one of the members of their team—hadn't lost their home, or knew somebody that did." When the hospital reopened, volunteers poured pitchers of warm water over the hands of the returning healthcare workers, while saying a blessing—a particularly poignant form of cleansing when surrounded by charred homes and ash. "That, to me, was a really crystallized example of how the volunteers were meeting the staff at a time when we were all very stressed, to have a very simple healing ritual," Dougherty said. Many of the managers also took up the practice, blessing the hands of their staff as the Threshold Choir sang at the entrance. "So you have them getting their hands blessed, you have these singers singing these beautiful messages of love and kindness and resiliency," he said. "I still have staff mention that, how moving it was."

While clinicians receive essential support from volunteers and non-clinical staff, management and administrative officials who are willing to step out from behind closed office doors to demonstrate appreciation can be equally, or even more, crucial. Sometimes it's as simple as blessing the hands of one's staff. At other times, it's listening and responding to a need for better benefits and pay, or reorganizing poorly functioning administrative procedures. Many less-visible clinical staff say they would benefit from being given time to grieve and process patient deaths, while all deserve to be included in debriefing from traumatic patient encounters. Support staff and volunteers who buttress doctors and nurses, and who keep healthcare institutions running smoothly, also need understanding, support, and appreciation for the essential roles that they play.

Conclusion:
Where to Next?

When I began conceptualizing this book in January 2020, the first COVID-19 cases were just emerging in China. By the end of that month, Wuhan was under quarantine, the first confirmed COVID-19 case had appeared in the US, and the World Health Organization had issued a global health emergency. Still, at that point, US healthcare workers had no way of anticipating what would emerge—more than half a million deaths across the country, school closures, lengthy social distancing measures. They had no way of knowing that we, as a society, would be directly confronted with the death, grief, and suffering we had tried so hard to avoid. Healthcare organizations were sometimes overwhelmed with patients; PPE shortages caused widespread anxiety; and family members were barred from their loved ones' bedsides, placing an even heavier burden on clinicians. Hospitals saw dramatic reductions in income as they temporarily halted services; many doctors, nurses, and other medical staff were severely overworked, while others lost their jobs.

The COVID-19 pandemic not only forced us to confront our existential denial of death, but it also unveiled the immense challenges inherent in the US medical system and their devastating impact on healthcare workers' mental health and emotional well-being. Medical personnel became more vocal about the lack of proper protection, impossible patient-staff ratios, and other failures of institutional support. Many were warned not to do so; others were fired. Lorna Breen, an emergency physician in New York who felt unable to do enough for her patients and feared licensing repercussions if she were to seek mental health services, committed suicide. Others struggled on, shouldering a heightened burden of grief and trauma—one that experts warned would result in widespread mental health challenges, burnout, and abdication from the profession, right at a time when it is facing massive workforce shortages. While there was an annual increase of 18 percent in applicants to medical school for the 2021–2022 academic year—due, in part, to relaxed criteria during the pandemic—the number of slots hadn't changed. There was still a massive deficit of healthcare workers required to meet the needs of a rapidly aging US population.

Meanwhile, the pandemic exposed the unequal burden of suffering shouldered by minorities in the nation's healthcare system—and society at large. Longstanding health disparities stemming from ongoing systemic racism and neglect were made visible as minority populations suffered disproportionately high numbers of infection, hospitalization, and death. Asian Americans blamed for the virus were targeted by hate crimes. And less visible frontline workers such as EVS workers, orderlies, and CNAs—many of whom were people of color—suffered from heightened exposure and died in greater numbers, as did those providing other forms of essential services.

So, what can be done? Terry Fulmer, president of the New York-based John A. Hartford Foundation, advocates for the federal government to fund scholarships, loan programs, and clinical internships to boost the medical workforce, as well as strengthen the Medicare Trust Fund (which the Congressional Budget Office predicted in September 2020 would be exhausted by 2024) and make better use of public Medicare dollars. "Firstly, you have to acknowledge [burnout] and really deal with the immediate trauma that the workforce has experienced over COVID," Fulmer said. "At least 3,000 healthcare professionals have died because of the pandemic. So you have to acknowledge that and understand that it's terrifying." In addition to boosting the workforce, Fulmer said, the US medical system needs to take action to rectify longstanding failures by providing better wages and benefits to CNAs, home health aides, nurses, LPNs, and other direct care workers. "You can give them free meals at work," she said. "You can provide their uniforms. You can provide free childcare. You can provide free transportation to and from work. That will all pay for itself in the quality of care." Finally, embracing telehealth will provide older adults with better access to healthcare while also reducing strain on clinicians, she said. Like Adam Gaffney, the former president of Physicians for a National Health Program, Fulmer supports a transition to Medicare for All or a single payer healthcare system that will both reduce burden on clinicians and provide more widespread access to care. "What we need to do is look at our deeply flawed, chronically underfunded way in which we take care of people," she said.

Healthcare is just one of the numerous US systems—along with social services and housing, among others—that the COVID-19 pandemic revealed to be severely lacking in humanity. While the Trump administration's initial response to the pandemic was woefully inadequate, healthcare workers have been dealing with the fallout of a detached and uncaring system for decades. The widespread lack of support for grief and trauma extends well beyond patient deaths and medical trauma to unrealistic work hours and schedules; escalating workplace violence; bullying; and other forms of mismanagement and abuse. Fortunately, the pandemic also highlighted the approaches that are working. Johns Hopkins' Resilience in Stressful Events (RISE) peer support program saw a dramatic increase in use of its services; institutions began offering more regular—and accessible—debriefings; and both individuals and healthcare organizations started acknowledging the importance of recognizing and addressing the impact of grief and trauma. Meanwhile, heartbreaking developments such as Breen's suicide highlighted the need for healthcare institutions to ensure private and confidential access to psychological and psychiatric care, and for state licensing boards to limit questions around mental health to those that are noninvasive, relevant, and compliant with the Americans with Disabilities Act.

Integrating grief and trauma for healthcare workers must begin in training and continue as an essential component throughout their careers—including varied offerings such as Schwartz Rounds, International Critical Incident Stress Foundation (ICISF) interventions, debriefings, coaching, and confidential and nonpunitive access to mental health services. No matter how much healthcare organizations might wish otherwise, there is no single solution—no silver bullet, no magic wand. Self-care trainings can be helpful, but they should be provided on paid workdays and acknowledge time constraints and other issues. Most importantly, such approaches simply cannot replace the need for widespread governmental, systemic, and institutional reform; improved staff support; and more reasonable work schedules, implemented with direct feedback from healthcare workers at all levels. More often than not, staff recognition is reduced to a pizza party or a coffee mug—minimal gestures that fail to recognize or address the traumatizing and grief-inducing circumstances they confront on a daily basis. Such token measures won't be enough. Catherine Sonquist, a family medicine physician and professor who's worked with the same cohort of students through medical school and residency in California, firmly believes that they will either change the system to make it more compassionate—or leave. "Healthcare is kind of like domestic violence, where people stay because we love healthcare and we love our patients but it's really very abusive," she told me. "There needs to be a fundamental reworking of the healthcare system; it needs to be overhauled. And if not, the crisis is going to be unparalleled."

Writing this book during a global pandemic has been a surreal experience, establishing a unique window into the challenges and sufferings of US healthcare workers at all levels of a malfunctioning system. Having absorbed this view, perhaps we can make the adjustments necessary to better support one another; to move toward a future that is more sustainable, more just. Not only for healthcare workers, but for all of us who will inevitably fall ill, suffer, and die—hopefully, with the best assistance possible at our bedsides. While the pandemic has made Americans more willing to accept the reality of their deaths—a 2021 survey found that 56 percent had engaged in end-of-life conversations, reflecting an increase of 24 percent from 2018—there is still much that we, as a society, refuse to acknowledge or address. What will those deaths look like? Where are our tax dollars going? How can we best prepare for a rapidly growing gray population? Are we treating our elders with dignity and respect? Is our current approach sustainable? In early 2020, when I first penned the introduction to this book—ending with the words "we're all in this together"—I couldn't have known that those very words would become a national catchphrase; a call to arms. I couldn't have imagined that a global pandemic would draw healthcare workers into the spotlight, while highlighting the systemic failings and burden of grief and trauma they must endure. Now, at least, we know where we are. "Where to next?" is an open question.

Notes

Introduction

p. 1. **life-changing article:** Kira Salak, "Places of Darkness: Africa's Mountain Gorillas and the War in Congo," *National Geographic Adventure*, 2004, http://www.kirasalak.com/Darkness.html.

p. 2. **1969 book:** Elisabeth Kübler-Ross, *On Death and Dying: What the Dying Have to Teach Doctors, Nurses, Clergy and Their Own Families* (New York: Scribner, 1997), 27–40, Kindle.

p. 2. **common for physicians:** Mark Siegler, "Recollections of Dr. Elisabeth Kübler-Ross at the University of Chicago (1965–70)," *The American Journal of Bioethics* 19, no. 12 (2019): 1–2, https://doi.org/10.1080/1526516 1.2019.1674550.

p. 3. **a small study:** Y. Dor-Ziderman, A. Lutz, and A. Goldstein, "Prediction-Based Neural Mechanisms for Shielding the Self from Existential Threat," *NeuroImage* 202, no. 116080 (November 15, 2019), https://doi.org/10.1016/j.neuroimage.2019.116080.

p. 3. **Freud wrote:** Sigmund Freud, "Thoughts for the Times on War and Death" in *The Standard Edition of the Complete Psychological Works of Sigmund Freud*, Vol. 14 (London: Hogarth Press, 1957), 289.

Chapter 1

p. 8. **satirical novel:** Samuel Shem, *The House of God* (New York: Berkley Books, 2010), 27, 37, Kindle.

p. 8. **a 2018 analysis:** Yi-Jung Tung, Kenneth K. H. Lo, Roger C. M. Ho, and Wai San Wilson Tam, "Prevalence of Depression among Nursing Students: A Systematic Review and Meta-analysis," *Nurse Education Today* 63 (April 2018): 119–129, https://doi.org/10.1016/j.nedt.2018.01.009.

p. 8 **In the clinical setting:** Darlene Del Prato, Esther Bankert, Patricia Grust, and Joanne Joseph, "Transforming Nursing Education: A Review of Stressors and Strategies That Support Students' Professional Socialization," *Advances in Medical Education and Practice* 2 (2011): 109–116, https://doi.org/10.2147/AMEP.S18359.

p. 8 **Negative or unsupportive relationships:** Dalton Henderson, Kerry A. Sewell, and Holly Wei, "The Impacts of Faculty Caring on Nursing Students' Intent to Graduate: A Systematic Literature Review," *International Journal of Nursing Sciences* 7, no. 1 (January 2020): 105–111, https://doi.org/10.1016/j.ijnss.2019.12.89.

p. 8 **Forty-four percent:** Leslie Kane, "Medscape National Physician Burnout, Depression and Suicide Report 2019," Medscape, January 16, 2019, https://www.medscape.com/slideshow/2019-lifestyle-burnout-depression-6011056.

p. 8 **Nearly a quarter:** Meredith Mealer, Jacqueline Jones, Julia Newman, Kim K. McFann, Barbara Rothbaum, and Marc Moss, "The Presence of Resilience Is Associated with a Healthier Psychological Profile in Intensive Care Unit (ICU) Nurses: Results of a National Survey," *International Journal of Nursing Studies* 49, no. 3 (March 2012): 292–299, https://doi.org/10.1016/j.ijnurstu.2011.09.015.

p. 9 **both nurses:** Judy Davidson, James Proudfoot, Kelly Lee, Garni Terterian, and Sidney Zisook, "A Longitudinal Analysis of Nurse Suicide in the United States (285–2016) with Recommendations for Action," *Worldviews on Evidence-Based Nursing* 17, no. 1 (2020): 6–15, https://doi.org/10.1111/wvn.12419.

p. 9 **and emergency medical technicians:** Neil Vigil, Andrew R. Grant, Octavio Perez, Robyn N. Blust, Vatsal Chikani, and Tyler F. Vadeboncoeur, "Death by Suicide—The EMS Profession Compared to the General Public," *Prehospital Emergency Care* 23, no. 3 (2019): 340–345, https://doi.org/10.1080/10903127.2018.1514090.

p. 9 **An estimated three hundred to four hundred physicians:** Pauline Anderson, "Physicians Experience Highest Suicide Rate of Any Profession," Medscape Medical News, May 7, 2018, https://www.medscape.com/viewarticle/896257.

p. 9 **Many factors:** Kane, "Burnout, Depression and Suicide Report 2019."

p. 9 **A 2017 study:** Leeat Granek, L. Barbera, O. Nakash, M. Cohen, and M. K. Krzyzanowska, "Experiences of Canadian Oncologists with Difficult

Patient Deaths and Coping Strategies Used," *Current Oncology* 24, no. 4 (2017): 277–284, https://doi.org/10.3747/co.24.3527.

p. 9 **previous research:** Leeat Granek, Richard Tozer, Paolo Mazzotta, Aliya Ramjaun, and Monika Krzyzanowska, "Nature and Impact of Grief Over Patient Loss on Oncologists' Personal and Professional Lives," *Archives of Internal Medicine* 172, no. 12 (2012): 964–966, https://doi.org/10.191/archinternmed.2012.1426.

p. 9 **US healthcare system:** "Timeline: History of Health Reform in the U.S.," Kaiser Family Foundation, accessed June 1, 2021, https://www.kff.org/wp-content/uploads/2011/03/5-02-13-history-of-health-reform.pdf.

p. 9 **many clinicians report:** Interviews with author, various dates.

p. 10 **series of books:** Sherry Lynn Jones, *Confessions of a Trauma Junkie: My Life as a Nurse Paramedic* (Ann Arbor: Modern History Press, 2017), Part I, Kindle.

p. 11 **doctoral dissertation for Walden University:** Sherry Lynn Jones, "Nurses' Occupational Trauma Exposure, Resilience, and Coping Education" (PhD diss., Walden University, 2016), https://scholarworks.waldenu.edu/dissertations/2360/.

p. 11 **psychologists define:** "Building Your Resilience," American Psychological Association, 2012, https://www.apa.org/topics/resilience.

p. 13 **Between 2000 and 2001:** Jennifer Rhodes-Kropf, Sharon Carmody, Deborah Seltzer, Ellen Redinbaugh, Nina Gadmer, Susan Block, and Robert Arnold, "'This Is Just Too Awful; I Just Can't Believe I Experienced That . . .': Medical Students' Reactions to Their 'Most Memorable' Patient Death," *Academic Medicine* 80, no. 7 (2005): 634–640, https://doi.org/10.1097/00001888-200507000-00005.

p. 13 **a separate study:** Ellen M. Redinbaugh, Amy M. Sullivan, Susan D. Block, Nina M. Gadmer, Matthew Lakoma, Ann M. Mitchell, Deborah Seltzer, Jennifer Wolford, and Robert M. Arnold, "Doctors' Emotional Reactions to Recent Death of a Patient: Cross Sectional Study of Hospital Doctors," *British Medical Journal* 327 (2003): 185, https://doi.org/10.1136/bmj.327.7408.185.

p. 13 **Treatment can turn:** "Radiation Therapy to the Head and Neck," Memorial Sloan Kettering Cancer Center, accessed June 1, 2021, https://www.mskcc.org/cancer-care/patient-education/radiation-therapy-head-and-neck.

p. 14 ***hidden curriculum:*** Philip Jackson, *Life in Classrooms* (New York: Holt, Rinehart & Winston, 1968), p. 33–35.

p. 14 **examples can include:** Lindsay Kalter, "Navigating the Hidden Curriculum in Medical School," Association of American Medical Colleges, July 30, 2019, https://www.aamc.org/news-insights/navigating-hidden-curriculum-medical-school.

p. 14 *pimping:* Frederick Brancati, "The Art of Pimping," *The Journal of the American Medical Association* 262, no. 1 (1989): 89–90, https://doi.org/10.1001/jama.1989.03430010101039.

p. 14 **"What role do prostaglandins . . .":** Brancati, "Art of Pimping," 89–90.

p. 15 **"What are the three signs . . .":** Abraar Karan, "Medical Students Need to Be Quizzed, but 'Pimping' Isn't Effective," STAT, February 3, 2017, https://www.statnews.com/2017/02/03/medical-students-pimping-testing-knowledge/.

p. 15 **40 percent of medical students:** "Medical School Graduation Questionnaire," Association of American Medical Colleges, July 2020, 38, https://www.aamc.org/media/46851/download.

p. 15 **repeat the cycle:** Christine Wiebe, "Medical Student 'Hazing' Is Unhealthy and Unproductive," Medscape, June 16, 2007, https://www.medscape.com/viewarticle/557598.

p. 15 **A study of AAMC data:** Katherine A. Hill, Elizabeth A. Samuels, Cary P. Gross, Mayur M. Desai, Nicole Sitkin Zelin, Darin Latimore, Stephen J. Hunt, Laura D. Cramer, Ambrose H. Wong, and Dowin Boatright, "Assessment of the Prevalence of Medical Student Mistreatment by Sex, Race/Ethnicity, and Sexual Orientation," *JAMA Internal Medicine* 180, no. 5 (2020): 653–665, https://doi.org/10.1001/jamainternmed.2020.0030.

p. 15 **women now graduate:** "Medical School Graduation Questionnaire," 5.

p. 15 **still experience:** Hill et al., "Prevalence of Medical Student Mistreatment," 653–665.

p. 15 **limited maternity leave:** Kirti Magudia, Alexander Bick, Jeffery Cohen, Thomas S. C. Ng, Debra Weinstein, Christina Magurian, and Reshma Jagsi, "Childbearing and Family Leave Policies for Resident Physicians at Top Training Institutions," *The Journal of the American Medical Association* 320, no. 22 (2018): 2372–2374, https://doi.org/10.1001/jama.2018.14414.

p. 15 **1998 classic,** Joan Cassell *The Woman in the Surgeon's Body* (Boston: Harvard University Press, 2000), Ch. 5, Kindle.

p. 15 **Racial discrimination:** Hill et al., ""Prevalence of Medical Student Mistreatment," 653–665.

p. 15 **little recourse:** Abraar Karan, "Why I Said Nothing When My Med School Professor Made Racist Remarks," WBUR, January 22, 2020, https://www.wbur.org/cognoscenti/2020/01/22/racial-harassment-doctor-medical-school-hospital-abraar-karan.

p. 16 **Studies have shown:** Liselotte N. Dyrbye, Colin P. West, Daniel Satele, Sonja Boone, Litjen Tan, Jeff Sloan, and Tait Shanafelt, "Burnout Among U.S. Medical Students, Residents, and Early Career Physicians Relative to the General U.S. Population," *Academic Medicine* 89, no. 3 (March 2014): 443–451, https://doi.org/10.1097/ACM.0000000000000134.

p. 16 **The American Medical Student Association:** "Report 6 of the Council on Medical Education," American Medical Association, 2019, https://www.ama-assn.org/system/files/2019-07/a19-cme-6.pdf.

p. 16 **an analysis of medical residency deaths:** Nicholas A. Yaghmour, Timothy P. Brigham, Thomas Richter, Rebecca S. Miller, Ingrid Philibert, Dewitt C. Baldwin, and Thomas J. Nasca, "Causes of Death of Residents in ACGME-Accredited Programs 2000 through 2014: Implications for the Learning Environment," *Academic Medicine* 92, no. 7 (2017): 976–983, https://doi.org/10.1097/ACM.0000000000001736.

p. 16 **began to lose interest:** Alison Cesarz, "Shining a Light on Medical School and Resident Depression," in-House, May 2, 2019, https://in-housestaff.org/shining-a-light-on-medical-student-and-resident-depression-1390.

p. 17 **More than a quarter:** Douglas A. Mata, Marco A. Ramos, Narinder Bansal, Rida Khan, Constance Guille, Emanuele Di Angelantonio, and Srijan Sen, "Prevalence of Depression and Depressive Symptoms Among Resident Physicians," *The Journal of the American Medical Association* 314, no. 22 (2015): 2373–2383, https://doi.org/10.1001/jama.2015.15845.

p. 17 **up from nearly 42 percent:** Srijan Sen, Henry R. Kranzler, John H. Krystal, Heather Speller, Grace Chan, Joel Gelernter, and Constance Guille, "A Prospective Cohort Study Investigating Factors Associated with Depression During Medical Internship," *Archives of General Psychiatry* 67, no. 6 (2010): 557–565, http://doi.org/10.1001/archgenpsychiatry.2010.41.

p. 17 **more likely to experience depression:** Karina Pereira-Lima, Rahael R. Gupta, Constance Guille, and Srijan Sen, "Residency Program Factors Associated with Depressive Symptoms in Internal Medicine Interns: A Prospective Cohort Study," *Academic Medicine* 94, no. 6 (June 2019): 869–875, https://doi.org/10.1097/ACM.0000000000002567.

p. 18 **Since 2003:** "The ACGME's Approach to Limit Resident Duty Hours 12 Months After Implementation: A Summary of Achievements,"

Accreditation Council for Graduate Medical Education, accessed June 1, 2021, https://www.acgme.org/Portals/0/PFAssets/Publications -Papers/dh_dutyhoursummary2003-04.pdf.

p. 18 **with the caveat:** "Common Program Requirements," Accreditation Council for Graduate Medical Education, effective July 1, 2011, https://www.acgme.org/Portals/0/PDFs/Common_Program_Requirements_07012011[2].pdf.

p. 18 **her intern year:** Frances Southwick, *Prognosis Poor: One Doctor's Personal Account of the Beauty and the Perils of Modern Medical Training* (n.p.: Book-Baby, 2015), Kindle.

p. 19 **the World Medical Association:** Ramin Walter Parsa-Parsi, "The Revised Declaration of Geneva: A Modern-Day Physician's Pledge," *The Journal of the American Medical Association* 318, no. 20 (2017): 1971–1972, https://doi.org/10.1001/jama.2017.16230.

p. 23 **A 2017 study of oncologists:** Leeat Granek, Merav Ben-David, Ora Nakash, Michal Cohen, Lisa Barbera, Samuel Ariad, and Monika K. Krzyzanowska, "Oncologists' Negative Attitudes towards Expressing Emotion over Patient Death and Burnout," *Supportive Care in Cancer* 25 (2017): 1607–1614, https://doi.org/10.1007/s00520-016-3562-y.

Chapter 2

p. 28 *Grief* **can be defined:** Christine A. Bruce, "Helping Patients, Families, Caregivers, and Physicians, in the Grieving Process," *The Journal of the American Osteopathic Association* 107, no. 7, (2007): ES33–ES40, https://www.degruyter.com/document/doi/10.7556/jaoa.2007.20039/html.

p. 28 **often involving:** APA Dictionary of Psychology, s.v. "Grief," American Psychological Association, accessed June 1, 2021, https://dictionary .apa.org/grief.

p. 28 **medical professionals retain vivid memories:** Interviews with author, various dates.

p. 32 **who coined the term:** "Disenfranchised Grief." Paper presented to a symposium on Death Education of the Foundation of Thalantology, New York, April 25, 1985, http://drkendoka.com/privacy-policy/.

p. 32 *disenfranchised grief:* K. J. Doka, "Disenfranchised Grief in Historical and Cultural Perspective," in M. S. Stroebe, R. O. Hansson, H. Schut, and W. Stroebe (Eds.) *Handbook of Bereavement Research and Practice: Advances in Theory and Intervention* (n.p.: American Psychological Association, 2008), 223–240, accessed June 1, 2021, https://doi.org/10.1037/14498-011.

p. 34 **viral LinkedIn post:** Louis M. Profeta, "I'll Look at Your Facebook Profile Before I Tell Your Mother You're Dead," LinkedIn, October 13, 2018, https://www.linkedin.com/pulse/ill-look-your-facebook-profile -before-i-tell-mother-youre-profeta-md/.

p. 37 **more than seventeen thousand oncologists:** Center for Workforce Studies, "2012 Physician Specialty Data Book," Association of American Medical Colleges, November 2012, 12, https://www.aamc.org/media/33486/download.

p. 37 **VitalTalk has trained:** Anthony Back, interview with author, July 20, 2020.

p. 38 **"Serious Illness Conversation Guide":** "Serious Illness Conversation Guide," Ariadne Labs and Dana-Farber Cancer Center, accessed September 19, 2021, https://www.ariadnelabs.org/wp-content/uploads /2017/05/SI-CG-2017-04-21_FINAL.pdf.

p. 39 **"integrated conclusion of care":** Alexandra Jabr, "It's Complicated: Grief and the First Responder," EMS World, October 1, 2019, https://www .emsworld.com/article/1223276/its-complicated-grief-and-first-responder.

p. 40 **more than a third:** "Medical School Graduation Questionnaire," Association of American Medical Colleges, July 2020, 3, https://www.aamc. org/media/46851/download.

p. 41 **were twenty times more likely:** Miriam Jordan and Richard A. Oppel, Jr. "For Latinos and Covid-19, Doctors Are Seeing an 'Alarming' Disparity," *New York Times*, May 7, 2020, https://www.nytimes.com/2020/05/07 /us/coronavirus-latinos-disparity.html.

p. 44 **the US Census total:** Tina Norris, Paula L. Vines, and Elizabeth M. Hoeffel, "The American Indian and Alaska Native Population: 2010," US Census Bureau, January 2012, 3, https://www.census.gov /history/pdf/c2010br-10.pdf.

p. 44 **a mere 0.2 percent:** "Diversity in Medicine: Facts and Figures 2019," Association of American Medical Colleges, 2019, https://www.aamc .org/data-reports/workforce/interactive-data/figure-2-percentage -applicants-us-medical-schools-race/ethnicity-alone-academic-year -2018-2019.

p. 44 **applicants of Hispanic:** "Quick Facts," US Census Bureau, July 1, 2019, https://www.census.gov/quickfacts/fact/table/US/PST045219.

p. 45 ***moral distress:*** Andrew Jameton, *Nursing Practice: The Ethical Issues* (Englewood Cliffs: Prentice-Hall, 1984), 6.

p. 45 **since been broadened:** Carina Fourie, "Who Is Experiencing What Kind of Moral Distress? Distinctions for Moving from a Narrow to a Broad Definition of Moral Distress," *AMA Journal of Ethics* 19, no. 6 (2017): 578–584, https://doi.org/10.1001/journalofethics.2017.19.6.nlit1-1706.

p. 47 **healthcare workers have reported:** "Safety and Health Topics/ Healthcare," Occupational Safety and Health Administration, US Department of Labor, accessed June 1, 2021, https://www.osha.gov /SLTC/healthcarefacilities/.

p. 47 **have some of the highest rates:** "Survey of Occupational Injuries and Illness Data," SNR01, US Bureau of Labor Statistics, 2018, https:// www.bls.gov/iif/soii-data.htm#summary.

p. 48 **personal protective equipment:** Susan R. Bailey, "Recurring PPE Short-ages Must Be Resolved Now," American Medical Association, August 26, 2020, https://www.ama-assn.org/about/leadership/recurring-ppe -shortages-must-be-resolved-now.

p. 48 **were furloughed or even lost their jobs:** Rachel Zimlich, "Covid-19 Staff Reductions," *Medical Economics* 97, no. 12 (2020): 54–59, https:// www.medicaleconomics.com/view/covid-19-staff-reductions.

p. 48 **700 healthcare worker deaths:** "Cases and Deaths among Healthcare Personnel," Covid Data Tracker, Centers for Disease Control and Pre-vention, accessed September 15, 2020, https://covid.cdc.gov/covid-data -tracker/#health-care-personnel.

p. 48 **an independent analysis:** Danielle Renwick and Shoshana Dubnow, "Exclusive: Over 900 Health Workers Have Died of COVID-19. And the Toll Is Rising," *The Guardian* and Kaiser Health News, August 11, 2020, https://khn.org/news/exclusive-over-900-health-workers-have-died-of -covid-19-and-the-toll-is-rising/.

p. 53 **three-quarters of occurring nonfatal assaults:** "Fact Sheet | Workplace Violence in Healthcare, 2018," Injuries, Illnesses, and Fatalities: US Bureau of Labor Statistics, April 2020, https://www.bls.gov/iif/oshwc /cfoi/workplace-violence-healthcare-2018.htm.

p. 53 **Nearly half of emergency physicians:** "ACEP Emergency Department Violence Poll Research Results," Marketing General Inc. for the Ameri-can College of Emergency Physicians, September 2018, https://www .emergencyphysicians.org/globalassets/files/pdfs/2018acep-emergency -department-violence-pollresults-2.pdf.

p. 53 **about 70 percent of emergency nurses:** "Workplace Violence," Emer-gency Nurses Association, accessed June 1, 2021, https://www.ena.org /practice-resources/workplace-violence.

p. 53 **have shot and killed patients:** Post-Tribune staff, "Security Guard's Shots Killed Co-worker, Patient in Munster Hospital Shooting, Prosecutor Says," *Chicago Tribune,* June 16, 2020, https://www.chicagotribune.com

/suburbs/post-tribune/ct-ptb-munster-community-hospital-shooting-st
-0617-20200616-256nfm2vgndyffsr6bu25id4qa-story.html.

p. 53 **one 2018 study:** Carmen R. Green, Wayne R. McCullough, and
Jamie D. Hawley, "Visiting Black Patients: Racial Disparities in Security
Standby Requests," *Journal of the National Medical Association* 110, no. 1
(February 2018): 37–43, https://doi.org/10.1016/j.jnma.2017.10.009.

p. 54 **published a 2018 paper:** Nursing Executive Center, "Rebuild the
Foundation for a Resilient Workforce," Advisory Board, August 8, 2018,
https://www.advisory.com/research/nursing-executive-center/white
-papers/2018/rebuild-the-foundation-for-a-resilient-workforce.

p. 55 **costing US hospitals:** Jill Van Den Bos, Nick Creten, Stoddard Dav-
enport, and Mason Roberts, "Cost of Community Violence to Hospitals
and Health Systems," Milliman Research Report for the American Hospital Association, July 26, 2017, https://www.aha.org/system/files/2018
-01/community-violence-report.pdf.

p. 55 **Data from the BLS:** Workplace Violence in Healthcare, 2018.

p. 55 **most of them:** "Emergency Department Violence Poll," 2018.

p. 55 **study of about 450 employees:** Judith Arnetz, Lydia Hamblin, Joel
Ager, Mark Luborsky, Mark J. Upfal, Jim Russell, and Lynnette Essen-
macher, "Underreporting of Workplace Violence: Comparison of Self-
Report and Actual Documentation of Hospital Incidents," *Workplace
Health and Safety* 63, no. 5 (2015): 200–210, https://doi
.org/10.1177/2165079915574684.

p. 55 **Contributing factors:** Arnetz et al., "Underreporting of Workplace
Violence," 200–210.

p. 55 **nurses have been warned:** Alexandra Robbins, *The Nurses: A Year of
Secrets, Drama, and Miracles with the Heroes of the Hospital* (New York: Work-
man Publishing Company, 2015), Ch. 3, Kindle.

p. 57 **commonly hazed and harassed:** "Medical School Graduation Questionnaire," July 2020.

p. 58 **Operating rooms are notorious:** Interviews with author, various dates.

p. 58 **cost expenditure:** Christopher P. Childers and Melinda Maggard-Gibbons,
"Understanding Costs of Care in the Operating Room," *JAMA Surgery* 153,
no. 4 (2018): e176233, https://doi.org/10.1001/jamasurg.2017.6233.

p. 59 **Male surgeons:** Joan Cassell, *The Woman in the Surgeon's Body* (Boston:
Harvard University Press, 2000), Ch. 5, Kindle.

p. 59 **A 1986 article:** Judith E. Meissner, "Nurses: Are We Eating Our
Young?" *Nursing* 16, no. 3 (1986): 51–53, https://pubmed.ncbi.nlm.nih
.gov/3633461/.

p. 60 **More than 180:** Renee Thompson, interview with author, August 5, 2020.

p. 61 **child bullies:** Joel Schwarz, "Violence in the Home Leads to Higher Rates of Childhood Bullying," University of Washington, September 12, 2006, https://www.washington.edu/news/2006/09/12/violence-in-the -home-leads-to-higher-rates-of-childhood-bullying/.

p. 62 **published one survey:** Alan H. Rosenstein and Michelle O'Daniel, "A Survey of the Impact of Disruptive Behaviors and Communication Defects on Patient Safety," *The Joint Commission Journal on Quality and Patient Safety* 34, no. 8 (August 2008): 464–471, https://doi.org/10.1016 /s1553-7250(08)34058-6.

p. 62 **anecdotal accounts:** Lev Raphael, "Warning: Doctors Can Be Bullies, Too," *Huffington Post,* updated December 23, 2017, https://www.huff-post.com/entry/saying-no-to-a-doctor-who-bullies-you_b_5a159335e4b0 09b331ad7661.

Chapter 4

p. 66 **affects more than 40 percent:** Leslie Kane, "Medscape National Physician Burnout, Depression and Suicide Report 2019," Medscape, January 16, 2019, https://www.medscape.com/slideshow/2019-lifestyle-burnout -depression-6011056.

p. 66 **"a long-term stress reaction . . .":** AMA, "What Should Be Done about the Physician Burnout Epidemic," Physician Health: American Medical Association, accessed June 1, 2021, https://www.ama-assn.org/practice-management/physician-health/what-should-be-done-about-physician -burnout-epidemic.

p. 66 **defines trauma:** APA Dictionary of Psychology, s.v. "trauma," American Psychological Association, accessed June 1, 2021, https://dictionary .apa.org/trauma.

p. 66 **Post-traumatic stress disorder:** DSM-5, "Posttraumatic Stress Disorder," *DSM-5* Fact Sheets, American Psychiatric Association, accessed June 1, 2021, https://www.psychiatry.org/psychiatrists/practice/dsm /educational-resources/dsm-5-fact-sheets.

p. 67 **In a 2012 study:** Meredith Mealer, Jacqueline Jones, Julia Newman, Kim K. McFann, Barbara Rothbaum, and Marc Moss, "The Presence of Resilience Is Associated with a Healthier Psychological Profile in Intensive Care Unit (ICU) Nurses: Results of a National Survey," *International Journal of Nursing Studies* 49, no. 3 (March 2012): 292–299, https:// doi.org/10.1016/j.ijnurstu.2011.09.015.

p. 68 **the only state that mandates:** "Nurse Staffing Advocacy," American Nurses Association, last updated July 2019, https://www.nursingworld .org/practice-policy/nurse-staffing/nurse-staffing-advocacy/.

p. 68 **many protested:** Kelly Gooch, "California Nurses Launch Statewide Protest against Waivers of Staffing Ratios," Becker's Hospital Review, updated February 2, 2021, https://www.beckershospitalreview.com/hr/california -nurses-launch-statewide-protest-against-waivers-of-staffing-ratios.html.

p. 68 **waived enforcement:** "Ratio Waiver Expires, Facilities Must Reapply," United Nurses Association of California, accessed June 1, 2021, https:// www.unacuhcp.org/ratio-waiver-expires-facilities-must-reapply/.

p. 69 **as Baby Boomers age:** America Counts Staff, "By 2030, All Baby Boomers Will Be Age 65 or Older," US Census Bureau, December 10, 2019, https://www.census.gov/library/stories/2019/12/by-2030-all-baby -boomers-will-be-age-65-or-older.html.

p. 69 **the average age:** Richard A. Smiley, Pamela Lauer, Cynthia Bienemy, Emilie Shireman, Kyrani A. Reneau, and Maryann Alexander, "The 2017 National Nursing Workforce Survey," *Journal of Nursing Regulation* 9, no. 3 (2018): S1–S88, https://doi.org/10.1016/S2155-8256 (18)30131-5.

p. 69 **approximately 200,000:** Elka Torpey, "Employment Outlook for Bachelor's-Level Occupations," Career Outlook, US Bureau of Labor Statistics, April 2018, https://www.bls.gov/careeroutlook/2018/article /bachelors-degree-outlook.htm#Healthcare%20and%20science.

p. 69 **more than 60,000:** "Rounds with Leadership: A 2020 View of the Nursing Workforce," American Association of Colleges of Nursing, January 29, 2020, https://www.aacnnursing.org/News-Information/News/View /ArticleId/24562/Rounds-with-Leadership-1-29-20.

p. 69 **a predicted deficit:** "New AAMC Report Confirms Growing Physician Shortage," Association of American Medical Colleges, June 26, 2020, https://www.aamc.org/news-insights/press-releases/new-aamc-report -confirms-growing-physician-shortage.

p. 69 **Congress placed a cap:** Jill Eden, Donald Berwick, and Gail Wilensky, eds., *Graduate Medical Education That Meets the Nation's Health Needs* (Washington, DC: National Academies Press, 2014), https://www.ncbi .nlm.nih.gov/books/NBK248024/.

p. 69 **the House:** Resident Physician Shortage Reduction Act of 2019, H.R. 1763, 116th Cong., March 14, 2019, https://www.congress.gov/bill /116th-congress/house-bill/1763?s=1&r=9.

p. 69 **and Senate:** Resident Physician Shortage Reduction Act of 2019, S. 348, 116th Cong., 1st sess., February 6, 2019, https://www.congress.gov /bill/116th-congress/senate-bill/348/text.

p. 69 **a suboptimal quarter:** "Graduate Medical Education: Training Tomorrow's Physician Workforce," Association of American Medical Colleges, accessed June 1, 2021, https://www.aamc.org/system/files/2020-06 /aamc-2020-workforce-projections-gme-training-workforce.pdf.

p. 69 **urology:** "Physician Workforce Planning and Graduate Medical Education," American Urological Association, accessed June 1, 2021, https://www.auanet.org/guidelines/physician-workforce-planning-and -graduate-medical-education.

p. 69 **Fifty-four percent:** Leslie Kane, "Medscape National Physician Burnout and Suicide Report 2020: The Generational Divide," Medscape, January 15, 2020, https://www.medscape.com/slideshow/2020 -lifestyle-burnout-6012460#4.

p. 70 **These figures updated:** Leslie Kane, "'Death by 1000 Cuts': Medscape National Physician Burnout and Suicide Report 2021," Medscape, January 22, 2021, https://www.medscape.com/slideshow/2021-lifestyle -burnout-6013456#2.

p. 71 **Female physicians:** Kim Templeton, Carol A. Bernstein, Javeed Sukhera, Lois Margaret Nora, Connie Newman, Helen Burstin, Constance Guille et al., "Gender-Based Differences in Burnout: Issues Faced by Women Physicians," National Academy of Medicine, May 30, 2019, https://doi.org/10.31478/201905a.

p. 72 **race and burnout:** Luis C. Garcia, Tait D. Shanafelt, Colin P. West, Christine A. Sinsky, Mickey T. Trockel, Laurence Nedelec, Yvonne A. Maldonado, Michael Tutty, Liselotte N. Dyrbye, and Magali Fassiotto, "Burnout, Depression, Career Satisfaction, and Work-Life Integration by Physician Race/Ethnicity," *JAMA Network Open* 3, no. 8 (2020): e2012762, http://doi.org/10.1001/jamanetworkopen.2020.12762.

p. 72 **race added an extra dimension:** Damon Tweedy, *Black Man in a White Coat: A Doctor's Reflections on Race and Medicine* (New York: Picador, 2015), Kindle.

p. 72 **The AAMC reported:** "Diversity in Medicine: Facts and Figures 2019," Association of American Medical Colleges, accessed June 1, 2021, https://www.aamc.org/data-reports/workforce/report/diversity -medicine-facts-and-figures-2019.

p. 73 **A landmark report:** Lina T. Kohn, Janet M. Corrigan, and Molla S. Donaldson, eds., *To Err Is Human: Building a Safer Health System* (Washington, DC: National Academy Press, 2000), https://doi.org/10.17226/9728.

p. 73 **a 2013 study:** John James, "A New, Evidence-based Estimate of Patient Harms Associated with Hospital Care," *Journal of Patient Safety* 9, no. 3 (2013): 122–128, https://doi.org/10.1097/PTS.0b013e3182948a69.

p. 74 **a short essay:** Albert Wu, "Medical Error: The Second Victim," *British Medical Journal* 320, no. 7237 (2000): 726–727, http://doi.org/10.1136 /bmj.320.7237.726.

p. 76 **jury reached a verdict:** Stacia Dearmin, "Experience Is Treacherous: An Intimate View of the Physician's Experience of Adverse Patient Outcomes and Malpractice Litigation," *Health Matrix: The Journal of Law-Medicine* 29, no. 1 (2019): 357–370, https://scholarlycommons.law.case .edu/cgi/viewcontent.cgi?article=1638&context=healthmatrix.

p. 76 **some 55:** Sandra Levy and Leslie Kane, "Medscape Malpractice Report 2017," Medscape, November 15, 2017, https://www.medscape .com/slideshow/2017-malpractice-report-6009206?faf=1#1.

p. 76 **75 percent:** Anupam B. Jena, Seth Seabury, Darius Lakdawalla, and Amitabh Chandra, "Malpractice Risk According to Physician Specialty," *The New England Journal of Medicine* 365 (2011): 629–636, https://doi .org/10.1056/NEJMsa1012370.

p. 77 **hundreds in the US:** Eileen Croke, "Nurses Negligence, and Malprac-tice: An Analysis Based on More Than 250 Cases against Nurses," *American Journal of Nursing* 103, no. 9 (September 2003): 54–63, http://doi .org/10.1097/00000446-200309000-00017.

p. 77 **book on medical error:** Danielle Ofri, *When We Do Harm: A Doctor Confronts Medical Error* (Boston: Beacon Press, 2020), p. 34–40; 152–153, Kindle.

p. 78 **Studies have shown:** Kristin E. Schleiter, "Difficult Patient-Physician Relationships and the Risk of Medical Malpractice Litigation," *AMA Journal of Ethics* 11, no. 3 (2009): 242–246, https://doi.org/10.1001 /virtualmentor.2009.11.3.hlaw1-0903.

p. 80 **A 2018 analysis:** Pauline Anderson, "Physicians Experience Highest Suicide Rate of Any Profession," Medscape Medical News, May 7, 2018, https://www.medscape.com/viewarticle/896257.

p. 80 **more than 860:** Pamela Wible, "Why 'Happy' Doctors Die by Suicide," Pamela Wible MD: America's Leading Voice for Ideal Medical Care, August 24, 2018, https://www.idealmedicalcare.org/why-happy-doctors -die-by-suicide/.

p. 80 **study in Arizona:** Neil Vigil, Andrew R. Grant, Octavio Perez, Robyn N. Blust, Vatsal Chikani, and Tyler F. Vadeboncoeur, "Death by Sui-cide—The EMS Profession Compared to the General Public," *Prehospital Emergency Care* 23, no. 3 (2019): 340–345, https://doi.org/10.1080/1090 3127.2018.1514090.

p. 82 **Studies are inconclusive:** Keith H. Berge, Marvin D. Seppala, and Agnes M. Schipper, "Chemical Dependency and the Physician," *Mayo Clinic Proceedings* 84, no. 7 (2009): 625–631, https://doi.org/10.1016 /S0025-6196(11)60751-9.

p. 83 **wasn't the first time:** Michael S. Weinstein, "Out of the Straitjacket," *The New England Journal of Medicine* 378 (2018) 793–795, https://doi .org/10.1056/NEJMp1715418.

Chapter 5

p. 88 **More than 650,000:** "Leading Causes of Death," National Center for Health Statistics, Centers for Disease Control and Prevention, accessed June 1, 2021, https://www.cdc.gov/nchs/fastats/leading-causes-of -death.htm.

p. 88 **of the 290,000-plus:** Lars W. Andersen, Mathias J. Holmberg, Katherine M. Berg, Michael W. Donnino, and Asger Granfeldt, "In-Hospital Cardiac Arrest: A Review," *The Journal of the American Medical Association* 321, no. 12 (2019): 1200–1210, https://doi.org/10.1001/jama.2019.1696.

p. 88 **less than 20 percent:** Uchenna R. Ofoma, Suresh Basnet, Andrea Berger, Lester Kirchner, and Saket Girotra, "Trends in Survival after In-Hospital Cardiac Arrest during Nights and Weekends," *Journal of the American College of Cardiology* 71, no. 4 (2018): 402–411, https://doi.org /10.1016/j.jacc.2017.11.043.

p. 89 **Transom radio piece:** Samuel Slavin, "Anatomy of A Code Blue," Transom, October 13, 2015, https://transom.org/2015/anatomy-of-a -code-blue/.

p. 90 **"the Medical Pause":** thepause.me, accessed August 31, 2021, https://thepause.me/.

p. 93 **required since the 1960s:** Masoud Kianpour, "Mental Health and Hospital Chaplaincy: Strategies of Self-Protection (Case Study: Toronto, Canada)," *Iranian Journal of Psychiatry and Behavioral Sciences* 7, no. 1 (2013): 69–77, https://www.ncbi.nlm.nih.gov/pmc/articles/PMC3939980/.

p. 98 **neuropsychiatric disorders:** "Mental Health and Mental Disorders," Office of Disease Prevention and Health Promotion, US Department of Health and Human Services, accessed June 1, 2021, https://www.healthy people.gov/2020/topics-objectives/topic/ mental-health-and-mental-disorders#2.

p. 98 **World Health Organization:** "The World Health Report : 2001 : Mental Health : New Understanding, New Hope," World Health Organization, 2001, 26, https://apps.who.int/iris/handle/10665/42390.

p. 98 **A 2016 Mayo Clinic study:** Liselotte N. Dyrbye, Colin P. West, Christine A. Sinsky, Lindsey E. Goeders, Daniel V. Satele, and Tail D. Shanafelt, "Medical Licensure Questions and Physician Reluctance to Seek Care for Mental Health Conditions," *Mayo Clinic Proceedings* 92, no. 10 (2017): 1486–1493, https://doi.org/10.1016/j.mayocp.2017.06.020.

p. 99 **a 2019 analysis:** Pamela Wible and Arianna Palermini, "Physician-Friendly States for Mental Health: A Comparison of Medical Licensing Board Applications," *Qualitative Research in Medicine and Healthcare* 3, no. 3 (2019): 107–119, https://doi.org/10.4081/qrmh.2019.8649.

p. 99 **a 2019 study:** Margaret J. Halter, Donna G. Rolin, Mona Adamaszek, Miles C. Ladenheim, and Bridet Frese Hutchens, "State Nursing Licensure Questions about Mental Illness and Compliance with the Americans with Disabilities Act," *Journal of Psychosocial Nursing and Mental Health Services* 57, no. 8 (2019) 17–22, https://doi.org/10.3928/02793695-20190405-02.

p. 99 **including California:** "Coming Soon: Changes to Medical Board Licensure Application," California Medical Association, May 28, 2019, https://www.cmadocs.org/newsroom/news/view/ArticleId/28075/Coming-Soon-Changes-to-medical-board-licensure-application.

p. 99 **and Florida:** Christine Sexton, "Florida Physician Boards Revamp Mental Health Questions," Health News Florida, October 2, 2020, https://health.wusf.usf.edu/health-news-florida/2020-10-02/florida-physician-boards-revamp-mental-health-questions.

p. 99 **controversial physician health programs:** Pauline Anderson, "Physician Health Programs: More Harm Than Good?," Medscape Medical News, August 19, 2015, https://www.medscape.com/viewarticle/849772.

p. 99 **published an article:** Melissa Freeman, "Nevertheless, I Have Persisted," *Qualitative Research in Medicine and Healthcare* 3, no. 3 (2019): 99–106, https://doi.org/10.4081/qrmh.2019.8638.

p. 99 **A lawyer for WPHP:** Kenneth Kagan, "Re: Washington Physicians Health Program," email to author, April 26, 2021.

p. 100 **positive participant stories:** "PHP Participant Stories," Federation of State Physician Health Programs, accessed June 1, 2021, https://www.fsphp.org/php-participant-stories.

p. 100 **as well as research:** "Research about PHPs and Health Professionals," Federation of State Physician Health Programs, accessed June 1, 2021, https://www.fsphp.org/research-about-phps-and-health-professionals.

p. 100 **"To avoid punishment":** Wible and Palermini, "Physician-Friendly States for Mental Health," 108.

p. 101 **one poll:** "Poll: Workplace Stigma, Fear of Professional Consequences Prevent Emergency Physicians from Seeking Mental Health
Care," American College of Emergency Physicians, October 26, 2020,
https://www.emergencyphysicians.org/article/mental-health/poll
-workplace-stigma-fear-of-professional-consequences-prevent-emergency
-physicians-from-seeking-mental-health-care.

Chapter 6

p. 105 **The gold standard:** C.P. West, L. N. Dyrbye, and T. D. Shanafelt,
"Physician Burnout: Contributors, Consequences and Solutions," *Journal
of Internal Medicine* 283, no. 6 (2018): 516–529, https://doi.org/10.1111
/joim.12752.

p. 105 **Maslach Burnout Inventory:** Christina Maslach and Susan Jackson, "The
Measurement of Experienced Burnout," *Journal of Occupational Behavior* 2,
no. 2 (1981): 99–113, https://doi.org/10.1002/job.4030020205.

p. 106 **as a senior resident:** "Physician Burnout with Dr. Tait Shanafelt,"
interview by Pavlos Tsantilas at Ninth Munich Vascular Conference,
Stanford Surgery, YouTube video, 25:59, December 18, 2019, https://
www.youtube.com/watch?v=ibkxmeeLWUc.

p. 106 **The resulting study:** Tait D. Shanafelt, Katherine A. Bradley, Joyce E.
Wipf, and Anthony L. Back, "Burnout and Self-Reported Patient Care
in an Internal Medicine Residency Program," *Annals of Internal Medicine*
136, no. 5 (2002): 358–367, https://doi.org/10.7326/0003-4819-136
-5-200203050-00008.

p. 106 **impact of a clinician's environment:** West, Dyrbye, and Shanafelt,
"Physician Burnout," 516–529.

p. 106 **high cost of physician turnover:** Shasha Han, Tait D. Shanafelt,
Christine A. Sinsky, Karim M. Awad, Liselotte N. Dyrbye, Lynne C.
Fiscus, Mickey Trockel, and Joel Goh, "Estimating the Attributable Cost
of Physician Burnout in the United States," *Annals of Internal Medicine*
170, no. 11 (2019): 784–790, https://doi.org/10.7326/M18-1422.

p. 106 **Dyrbye's work:** Liselotte N. Dyrbye, Matthew R. Thomas, F. Stand-
ford Massie, David V. Power, Anne Eacker, William Harper, Steven
Durning et al., "Burnout and Suicidal Ideation among U.S. Medical Students," *Annals of Internal Medicine* 149, no. 5 (2008): 334–341, https://
doi.org/10.7326/0003-4819-149-5-200809020-00008.

p. 106 **nearly a third of them:** Liselotte N. Dyrbye, Matthew R. Thomas, and
Tait D. Shanafelt, "Medical Student Distress: Causes, Consequences,

and Proposed Solutions," *Mayo Clinic Proceedings* 80, no. 12 (2005): 1613–1622, https://doi.org/10.4065/80.12.1613.

p. 106 **Other medical schools had:** Stuart J. Slavin, Debra L. Schindler, and John T. Chibnall, "Medical Student Mental Health 3.0: Improving Student Wellness through Curricular Changes," *Academic Medicine* 89, no. 4 (2014): 573–577, http://doi.org/10.1097/ACM.0000000000000166.

p. 107 **First- and second-year medical students:** Slavin, Schindler, and Chibnall, "Medical Student Mental Health 3.0," 573–577.

p. 107 **led to higher scores:** Slavin, Schindler, and Chibnall, "Medical Student Mental Health 3.0," 573–577.

p. 107 **Evaluations:** Slavin, Schindler, and Chibnall, "Medical Student Mental Health 3.0," 573–577.

p. 107 **sociologist Renée Fox:** Renée Fox, "Training for Uncertainty" in *The Student-Physician: Introductory Studies in the Sociology of Medical Education* (Cambridge: Harvard University Press, 1957): 208–209.

p. 107 **In February 2017:** Kevin Behrns, "Transforming Excellence in Academic Medicine," *Missouri Medicine* 115, no. 3 (2018): 203–205, https://www.ncbi.nlm.nih.gov/pmc/articles/PMC6140140/.

p. 108 **despite protests from students:** Sandra Jordan, "SLU Med Students Protest Dismissal of Dean, Dr. Stuart Slavin Takes Fall for Negative Accreditation Report," *St. Louis American*, May 15, 2017, http://www.stlamerican.com/news/local_news/slu-med-students-protest-dismissal-of-dean-dr-stuart-slavin-takes-fall-for-negative-accreditation/article_64ad0766-39bd-11e7-aac2-0796d83193d7.html.

p. 108 **cleared by the accrediting body:** Nancy Solomon, "Probation Lifted for SLU's Medical School," Saint Louis University, October 10, 2018, https://www.slu.edu/news/2018/october/lcme-probation-lifted.php.

p. 108 **AWARE:** Susan White, "ACGME Launches AWARE Well-Being Resources," Accreditation Council for Graduate Medical Education, December 4, 2019, https://acgme.org/Newsroom/Newsroom-Details/ArticleID/9786/ACGME-Launches-AWARE-Well-Being-Resources.

p. 109 **that Maslach identified:** Christina Maslach and Michael P. Leiter, "Understanding the Burnout Experience: Recent Research and Its Implications for Psychiatry," *World Psychiatry* 15, no. 2 (2016): 103–111, https://doi.org/10.1002/wps.20311.

p. 109 **"Penn Face":** Lucy Hu, "Penn Face Is a Part of Who We Are," *Daily Pennsylvanian*, September 26, 2017, https://www.thedp.com/article/2017/09/lucy-hu-penn-face-is-a-part-of-who-we-are.

p. 109 **"Duck Syndrome":** Tiger Sun, "Duck Syndrome and a Culture of Misery," *Stanford Daily,* January 31, 2018, https://www.stanforddaily.com/2018
/01/31/duck-syndrome-and-a-culture-of-misery/.

p. 110 **Another innovator:** Rachel Naomi Remen, *Kitchen Table Wisdom: Stories That Heal* (New York: Riverhead Books, 1996), Kindle.

p. 110 **"The Healer's Art,"** Rachel Naomi Remen MD: Remembering Your Power to Heal, accessed September 1, 2021, http://www.rachelremen
.com/learn/medical-education-work/the-healers-art/.

p. 110 **the professional liability crisis:** Deborah Lewis-Idema, "Medical Professional Liability and Access to Obstetrical Care: Is There a Crisis?" in Victoria Rostow and Roger Bulger, eds., *Medical Professional Liability and the Delivery of Obstetrical Care: Volume II, An Interdisciplinary Review* (Washington, DC: The National Academies Press, 1989), chap. 5, https://www
.ncbi.nlm.nih.gov/books/NBK218646/.

p. 111 **51.6 percent of students:** Elizabeth C. Lawrence, Martha L. Carvour, Christopher Camarata, Evangeline Andarsio, and Michael W. Rabow, "Requiring the Healer's Art Curriculum to Promote Professional Identify Formation among Medical Students," *Journal of Medical Humanities* 41 (2020): 531–541, https://doi.org/10.1007/s10912-020-09649-z.

p. 112 **the Stanford Model:** "The Stanford Model of Professional Fulfillment," Stanford Medicine, accessed June 1, 2021, https://wellmd
.stanford.edu/about/model-external.html.

p. 112 **New Mexico's licensing application:** Eileen Barrett, Elizabeth Lawrence, Daniel Waldman, and Heather Brislen, "Improving How State Medical Boards Ask Physicians about Mental Health Diagnoses: A Case Study from New Mexico," *Annals of Internal Medicine* 172, no. 9 (2020): 617–618, https://doi.org/10.7326/M19-3681.

p. 113 **the efficacy of the arts:** Salvatore Mangione, Chayan Chakraborti, Giuseppe Staltari, Rebecca Harrison, Allan R. Tunkel, Kevin T. Liou, Elizabeth Cerceo et al., "Medical Students' Exposure to the Humanities Correlates with Positive Personal Qualities and Reduced Burnout: A Multi-Institutional U.S. Survey," *Journal of General Internal Medicine* 33 (2018) 628–634, https://doi.org/10.1007/s11606-017-4275-8.

p. 113 **student wrote an article:** Michael Poulson, "At 18 Years Old, He Donated a Kidney. Now, He Regrets It.," *Washington Post,* October 2, 2016, https://www.washingtonpost.com/national/health-science/at-18
-years-old-he-donated-a-kidney-now-he-regrets-it/2016/09/30/cc9407d8
-5ff9-11e6-8e45-477372e89d78_story.html.

p. 114 **European and US urology residents:** Daniel Marchalik, Charlotte C. Goldman, Flippe F. L. Carvalho, Michele Talso, John H. Lynch, Francesco Espereto, Benjamin Pradere, Jeroen Van Besien, and Ross E. Krasnow, "Resident Burnout in USA and European Urology Residents: An International Concern," *BJU International* 124, no. 2 (2019): 349–356, https://doi.org/10.1111/bju.14774.

p. 114 **US palliative care providers:** Daniel Marchalik, Ariel Rodriguez, Amalia Namath, Ross Krasnow, Simone Obara, Jamie Padmore, and Hunter Groninger, "The Impact of Non-medical Reading on Clinician Burnout: A National Survey of Palliative Care Providers," *Annals of Palliative Medicine* 8, no. 4 (2019): 428–435, https://doi.org/10.21037/apm.2019.05.02.

p. 117 **the knitting intervention:** Lyndsay Anderson and Christina U. Gustavson, "The Impact of a Knitting Intervention on Compassion Fatigue in Oncology Nurses," *Clinical Journal of Oncology Nursing* 20, no. 1 (2016): 102–104, https://doi.org/10.1188/16.CJON.102-104.

p. 117 **Betsan Corkhill:** "Guide to Our Theories So Far," Stitchlinks, April 2008, http://www.stitchlinks.com/pdfsNewSite/research/Our%20theories%20so%20far%20New_%20unshuffled%20watermarked_4.pdf.

p. 118 **studies provided convincing evidence:** Liselotte N. Dyrbye, Tait D. Shanafelt, Priscilla R. Gill, Daniel V. Satele, and Colin P. West., "Effect of a Professional Coaching Intervention on the Well-Being and Distress of Physicians," *JAMA Internal Medicine* 179, no. 10 (2019): 1406–1414, https://doi.org/10.1001/jamainternmed.2019.2425.

p. 123 **physician mental health advocate:** Pamela Wible, *Physician Suicide Letters—Answered* (Oregon: Pamela Wible, MD, Publishing, 2016), Kindle.

Chapter 7

p. 127 **Carla Joinson**: Deborah Boyle, "Countering Compassion Fatigue: A Requisite Nursing Agenda," *Online Journal of Issues in Nursing* 16, no. 1 (2011): 2, https://pubmed.ncbi.nlm.nih.gov/21800933/.

p. 128 **in a medical sense:** Merriam-Webster online, s.v. "compassion fatigue," accessed June 1, 2021, https://www.merriam-webster.com/dictionary/compassion%20fatigue.

p. 128 **with *secondary traumatic stress*:** Charles Figley, *Compassion Fatigue: Coping with Secondary Traumatic Stress Disorder in Those Who Treat the Traumatized* (New York: Routledge, 1995).

p. 128 **state in their book:** Stephen Trzeciak and Anthony Mazzarelli, *Compassionomics: The Revolutionary Scientific Evidence That Caring Makes a Difference* (Pensacola: Studer Group, 2019), Introduction, Kindle.

p. 128 **depersonalization is a key indicator:** C.P. West, L. N. Dyrbye, and T. D. Shanafelt, "Physician Burnout: Contributors, Consequences and Solutions," *Journal of Internal Medicine* 283, no. 6 (2018): 516–529, https://doi.org/10.1111/joim.12752.

p. 131 **one dramatic example:** Trzeciak and Mazzarelli, *Compassionomics,* chap. 3, Kindle.

p. 134 **costs US health systems:** "The Business Case for Humanity in Healthcare," National Taskforce for Humanity in Healthcare, April 2018, https://www.vocera.com/public/pdf/NTHBusinessCase_final003.pdf.

p. 134 **millennial physicians:** Robert Nagler Miller, "Millennial Physicians Sound Off on State of Medicine Today," American Medical Association, March 27, 2017, https://www.ama-assn.org/practice-management/physician-health/millennial-physicians-sound-state-medicine-today.

p. 134 **high-paying specialties:** Keith L. Martin, "Medscape Physician Lifestyle and Happiness Report 2020: The Generational Divide," January 8, 2020, https://www.medscape.com/slideshow/2020-lifestyle-generational-6012424#4.

p. 134 **female physicians:** Leslie Kane, "Women Physicians 2020: The Issues They Care About," July 15, 2020, https://www.medscape.com/slideshow/2020-women-physicians-6013042?faf=1#2.

p. 134 **emergency doctors typically work:** James Dahle, "7 Reasons Why This Physician Works Half-Time," KevinMD.com, October 16, 2018, https://www.kevinmd.com/blog/2018/10/7-reasons-why-this-physician-works-half-time.html.

p. 135 **six hours charting:** Brian G. Arndt, John W. Beasley, Michelle D. Watkinson, Jonathan L. Temte, Wen-Jan Tuan, Christine A. Sinsky, and Valerie J. Gilchrist, "Tethered to the EHR: Primary Care Physician Workload Assessment Using EHR Event Log Data and Time-Motion Observations," *Annals of Family Medicine* 15, no. 5 (2017): 419–426, https://doi.org/10.1370/afm.2121.

p. 137 **five sources of hope:** Alphonsus Obayuwana, *The Five Sources of Human Hope: Mirror of Our Humanity* (Bloomington: iUniverse, 2012), chap. 2, Kindle.

p. 138 **thesis on hoop dancing:** Caroline Sánchez, Anna Valdez, and Lori Johnson, "Hoop Dancing to Prevent and Decrease Burnout and

Compassion Fatigue," *Journal of Emergency Nursing* 40, no. 4 (2014): 394–395, https://doi.org/10.1016/j.jen.2014.04.013.

p. 140 **first narrative medicine program:** Rita Charon, Sayantani DasGupta, Nellie Hermann, Craig Irvine, Eric R. Marcus, Edgar Rivera Colón, Danielle Spencer, and Maura Spiegel, "The Principles and Practice of Narrative Medicine," Columbia University Department of Medical Humanities and Ethics, accessed September 1, 2021, https://www.mhe.cuimc .columbia.edu/our-divisions/division-narrative-medicine/principles -and-practice-narrative-medicine.

p. 143 **Shackleton insisted:** Alfred Lansing, *Endurance: Shackleton's Incredible Voyage* (New York: Basic Books, 2014), chap. 1, Kindle.

Chapter 8

p. 146 **a corporate behemoth:** Marion Mass, "American Healthcare: Increasingly Corporate and Rapacious," Medpage Today, February 10, 2020, https://www.medpagetoday.com/publichealthpolicy/ healthpolicy/84795.

p. 146 **2020 Gallup poll:** Lydia Saad, "U.S. Ethics Ratings Rise for Medical Workers and Teachers," Gallup, December 22, 2020, https://news.gallup. com/poll/328136/ethics-ratings-rise-medical-workers-teachers.aspx.

p. 147 **the resulting paper:** Jamie Lynn Leslie and William Lonneman, "Promoting Trust in the Registered Nurse-Patient Relationship," *Home Healthcare Now* 34, no. 1 (2016): 38–42, https://doi.org/10.1097 /NHH.0000000000000322.

p. 148 **published several papers:** David H. Thom, Mark A. Hall, and L. Gregory Pawlson, "Measuring Patients' Trust in Physicians When Assessing Quality of Care," *Health Affairs* 23, no. 4 (2004): 124–132, https:// doi.org/10.1377/hlthaff.23.4.124.

p. 148 **US has been struggling:** "National Health Insurance—A Brief History of Reform Efforts in the U.S.," Focus on Health Reform: Kaiser Family Foundation, March 2009, 3–4, https://www.kff.org/wp-content /uploads/2013/01/7871.pdf.

p. 149 **millions of dollars:** Frank Campion, *The AMA and US Health Policy Since 1940* (Chicago: Chicago Review Press, 1984), 158.

p. 149 **Health Maintenance Organization Act:** "Implementation of the Health Maintenance Organization Act of 1973, as Amended," U.S. Government Accountability Office, March 3, 1978, https://www.gao.gov/products /105122.

p. 149 **managed care:** *Encyclopedia Britannica Online,* s.v. "Managed care," accessed June 1, 2021, https://www.britannica.com/topic/managed-care.

p. 149 **increasingly corporatized model:** Elisabeth Rosenthal, "Insurance Policy: How an Industry Shifted from Protecting Patients to Seeking Profit," Stanford Medicine, Spring 2017, https://stanmed.stanford.edu /2017spring/how-health-insurance-changed-from-protecting-patients -to-seeking-profit.html.

p. 149 **"Open Payments":** "Open Payments," US Centers for Medicare and Medicaid Services, accessed September 1, 2021, https://openpayments data.cms.gov/.

p. 150 **its own issues:** Cristobal Young and Xinxiang Chen, "Patients as Consumers in the Market for Medicine: The Halo Effect of Hospitality," *Social Forces* 99, no. 2 (2020): 504–531, https://doi.org/10.1093/sf/soaa007.

p. 150 **A national 2018 survey:** "The Future of Healthcare: A National Survey of Physicians," The Doctors Company, accessed September 1, 2021, https://www.thedoctors.com/about-the-doctors-company /newsroom/the-future-of-healthcare-survey/.

p. 150 **25 percent of hospital revenue:** David U. Himmelstein, Miraya Jun, Karine Chevreul, Alexander Geissler, Patrick Jeurissen, Sarah Thomson, Marie-Amelie Vinet, and Steffie Woolhandler, "A Comparison of Hospital Administrative Costs in Eight Nations: US Costs Exceed All Others by Far," *Health Affairs* 33, no. 9 (2014): 1586–1594, https://doi.org/10 .1377/hlthaff.2013.1327.

p. 151 **not allotted enough time:** Mark Linzer, Thomas R. Konrad, Jeffrey Douglas, Julia E. McMurray, Donald E. Pathman, Eric S. Williams et al., "Managed Care, Time Pressure, and Physician Job Satisfaction: Results from the Physician Worklife Study," *Journal of General Internal Medicine* 15, no. 7 (2000): 441–450, https://doi.org/10.1046/j.1525-1497.2000.05239.x.

p. 151 **Tuskegee:** "The U.S. Public Health Service Syphilis Study at Tuskegee," Centers for Disease Control and Prevention, accessed June 1, 2021, https://www.cdc.gov/tuskegee/index.html.

p. 151 **Marion Sims's experimentation:** Durrenda Ojanuga, "The Medical Ethics of the 'Father of Gynaecology', Dr. J Marion Sims," *Journal of Medical Ethics* 19, no. 1 (1993): 28–31, https://doi.org/10.1136/jme.19.1.28.

p. 152 **NMA task force:** Leon McDougle, "Advisory Statement on Federal Drug Administration's Emergency Use Authorization Approval for Pfizer and Moderna Vaccine," National Medical Association, December 21, 2020, https://www.nmanet.org/news/544970/NMA-COVID-19-Task -Force-on-Vaccines-and-Therapeutics.htm.

p. 152 **less than 80 percent:** Tarryn Mento, "Southeast San Diego COVID-19 Testing Site to Become Walk-In Location after High No-Show Rate," KPBS, June 22, 2020, https://www.kpbs.org/news/2020/jun/22/low-turnout-puts-state-covid-testing-site-risk-sou/.

p. 153 **his innovative approaches:** Adrian Owen, *Into the Gray Zone: A Neuroscientist Explores the Border between Life and Death* (New York: Scribner, 2017), Kindle.

p. 154 **now widely accepted:** Damian Cruse, Srivas Chennu, Camille Chatelle, Tristan A. Bekinschtein, Davinia Fernández-Espejo, John D. Pickard, Steven Laureys, and Adrian M. Owen, "Bedside Detection of Awareness in the Vegetative State: A Cohort Study," *The Lancet* 378, no. 9809 (2011): 2088–2094, https://doi.org/10.1016/S0140-6736(11)61224-5.

p. 154 **vegetative states may be misdiagnosed:** Caroline Schnakers, Audrey Vanhaudenhuyse, Joseph Giacino, Manfredi Ventura, Melanie Boly, Steve Majerus, Gustave Moonen, and Steven Laureys, "Diagnostic Accuracy of the Vegetative and Minimally Conscious State: Clinical Consensus versus Standardized Neurobehavioral Assessment," *BMC Neurology* 9, no. 35 (2009), https://doi.org/10.1186/1471-2377-9-35.

p. 156 **nearly 3 million traumatic brain injuries:** Alexis B. Peterson, Hong Zhou, Karen E. Thomas, Jill Daugherty, and Alexis B. Peterson, "Surveillance Report: Traumatic Brain Injury-Related Hospitalizations and Deaths by Age Group, Sex, and Mechanism of Injury," Centers for Disease Control and Prevention, 2016 and 2017, https://www.cdc.gov/traumaticbraininjury/pdf/TBI-surveillance-report-2016-2017-508.pdf.

p. 156 **denied rehab:** Tamar Ezer, Megan S. Wright, and Joseph J. Fins, "The Neglect of Persons with Severe Brain Injury in the United States: An International Human Rights Analysis," *Health and Human Rights Journal* 22, no. 1 (2020): 265–278, https://www.hhrjournal.org/2020/06/the-neglect-of-persons-with-severe-brain-injury-in-the-united-states-an-international-human-rights-analysis/.

p. 158 **experienced locked-in syndrome:** Jean-Dominique Bauby, *The Diving Bell and the Butterfly: A Memoir of Life in Death* (New York: Vintage, 1998), Kindle.

p. 160 **one told her mother:** Owen, *Into the Gray Zone*, chap. 10.

p. 160 **Bender Pape's earlier research:** Theresa Louise-Bender Pape, Joshua M. Rosenow, Monica Steiner, Todd Parrish, Ann Guernon, Brett Harton, Vijaya Patil et al., "Placebo-Controlled Trial of Familiar Auditory Sensory Training for Acute Severe Traumatic Brain Injury: A Preliminary Report," *Neurorehabilitation and Neural Repair* 29, no. 6 (2015): 537–547, https://doi.org/10.1177/1545968314554626.

p. 164 **J.D. Old Mouse:** "In Memory of Jay Dale Old Mouse, Age 53, of Busby," Stevenson & Sons Funeral Homes, accessed June 1, 2021, https://stevensonfuneralhomes.com/obituaries/j-d-oldmouse-age-53-of-lame-deer/.

p. 166 **one veteran named Tom:** Bessel van der Kolk, *The Body Keeps the Score: Brain, Mind and the Body in the Healing of Trauma* (New York: Penguin, 2014), chap. 1, Kindle.

Chapter 9

p. 170 **life review:** Mimi Jenko, Leah Gonzalez, and Mary Jane Seymour, "Life Review with the Terminally Ill," *Journal of Hospice & Palliative Nursing* 9, no. 3 (2007): 159–167, https://doi.org/10.1097/01.NJH.0000269995.98377.4d.

p. 170 **concept of hospice care:** "History of Hospice," National Hospice and Palliative Care Organization, accessed June 1, 2021, https://www.nhpco.org/hospice-care-overview/history-of-hospice/.

p. 170 **independently formed:** Joy Buck, "Policy and the Reformation of Hospice: Lessons from the Past for the Future of Palliative Care," *Journal of Hospice & Palliative Nursing* 13, no. 6 (2011): 35–43, https://doi.org/10.1097/NJH.0b013e3182331160.

p. 170 **Fifteen years after:** Cynthia Adams, "Dying with Dignity in America: The Transformational Leadership of Florence Wald," *Journal of Professional Nursing* 26, no. 2 (2010): 125–132, https://doi.org/10.1016/j.profnurs.2009.12.009.

p. 170 **more than 4,500:** "NHPCO Facts and Figures," National Hospice and Palliative Care Organization," August 20, 2020, p. 20.

p. 170 **hospice and palliative medicine:** "ABMS Subspecialty Certification in Hospice and Palliative Medicine," American Academy of Hospice and Palliative Medicine, accessed June 1, 2021, https://aahpm.org/certification/subspecialty-certification.

p. 171 **Americans age sixty-five:** America Counts Staff, "By 2030, All Baby Boomers Will Be Age 65 or Older," US Census Bureau, December 10, 2019.

p. 171 **life expectancy:** Wan He, Daniel Goodkind, and Paul Kowal, "An Aging World: 2015," US Census Bureau, March 2016, 35, https://www.census.gov/content/dam/Census/library/publications/2016/demo/p95-16-1.pdf.

p. 171 **focus group study:** Rebecca H. Lehto, Carrie Heeter, Jeffrey Forman, Tait Shanafelt, Arif Kamam, Patrick Miller, and Michael Paletta, "Hospice Employees' Perceptions of Their Work Environment: A Focus Group

Perspective," *International Journal of Environmental Research and Public Health* 17, no. 17 (2020): 6147, https://doi.org/10.3390/ijerph17176147.

p. 171 **die at home:** "NHPCO Facts and Figures," 15.

p. 171 **Americans state as their preference:** Liz Hamel, Bryan Wu, and Mollyann Brodie, "Views and Experiences with End-of-Life Medical Care in the U.S.," Kaiser Family Foundation, April 27, 2017, https://www.kff.org/report-section/views-and-experiences-with-end-of-life-medical-care-in-the-us-findings/.

p. 171 **Medicare only covers it:** "Hospice care," Medicare.gov, accessed June 1, 2021, https://www.medicare.gov/coverage/hospice-care.

p. 172 **Of the 1.1 million:** "NHPCO Facts and Figures," 15.

p. 172 **days that involved hospice care:** "NHPCO Facts and Figures," 17.

p. 172 **less than a month:** "NHPCO Facts and Figures," 12.

p. 173 **In a small study:** Angela Ghesquiere and Ariunsanaa Bagaajav, "'We Take Care of People; What Happens to Us Afterwards?': Home Health Aides and Bereavement Care in Hospice," *OMEGA – Journal of Death and Dying* 80, no. 4 (2018): 615–628, https://doi.org/10.1177/0030222818754668.

p. 180 **One study suggests:** Lori Montross-Thomas, Caroline Scheiber, Emily A. Meier, and Scott A. Irwin, "Personally Meaningful Rituals: A Way to Increase Compassion and Decrease Burnout among Hospice Staff and Volunteers," *Journal of Palliative Medicine* 19, no. 10 (2016): 1043–1050, https://doi.org/10.1089/jpm.2015.0294.

p. 182 **a national study:** Montross-Thomas et al., "Personally Meaningful Rituals," 1043–1050.

Chapter 10

p. 188 **clinical death was defined:** Ben Sarbey, "Definitions of Death: Brain Death and What Matters in a Person," *Journal of Law and the Biosciences* 3, no. 3 (2016): 743–752, https://doi.org/10.1093/jlb/lsw054.

p. 188 **Uniform Determination of Death Act:** National Conference of Commissioners on Uniform State Laws, "Uniform Determination of Death Act," accessed June 1, 2021, http://www.lchc.ucsd.edu/cogn_150/Readings/death_act.pdf.

p. 188 **new research:** Zvonimir Vrselja, Stefano G. Daniele, John Sibereis, Francesca Talpl, Yury M. Morozov, André M. M. Sousa, Brian S. Tanka et al., "Restoration of Brain Circulation and Cellular Function Hours Post-mortem," *Nature* 568 (2019): 336–343, https://www.nature.com/articles/s41586-019-1099-1.

p. 189 **irreversible brain injury:** Joseph J. Gallo, Joseph B. Straton, Michael J. Klag, Lucy A. Meoni, Daniel P. Sulmasy, Nae-yuh Wang, and Daniel E. Ford, "Life-Sustaining Treatments: What Do Physicians Want and Do They Express Their Wishes to Others?" *Journal of the American Geriatrics Society* 51, no. 7 (2003): 961–969, https://doi.org/10.1046/j.1365-2389.2003.51309.x.

p. 189 *palliative care* **was coined:** "Palliative Care McGill – History," McGill University, accessed June 1, 2021, https://www.mcgill.ca/palliativecare /about-us/history.

p. 189 **interview with McGill University:** Devon Phillips, "Balfour Mount," McGill University, accessed June 1, 2021, https://www.mcgill.ca /palliativecare/portraits-0/balfour-mount.

p. 189 **has since evolved:** Qiaohong Guo, Cynthia S. Jacelon, and Jenna L. Marquard, "An Evolutionary Concept Analysis of Palliative Care," *Journal of Palliative Care and Medicine* 2, no. 7 (2012): 1000127, https://doi .org/10.4172/2165-7386.1000127.

p. 190 **72 percent of US hospitals:** "America's Care of Serious Illness," Center to Advance Palliative Care, 2019, 6, https://reportcard.capc .org/wp-content/uploads/2020/05/CAPC_State-by-State-Report -Card_051120.pdf.

p. 190 **only physicians:** Jean Acevedo, "Documentation & Coding Handbook: Palliative Care," Acevedo Consulting Inc., 2019, 1, https://www .chcf.org/wp-content/uploads/2019/05/DocumentationCoding HandbookPalliativeCare.pdf.

p. 191 **on a research paper:** Emily L. Aaronson, Laura Petrillo, Mark Stoltenberg, Juliet Jacobsen, Erica Wilson, Jason Bowman, Kei Ouchi et al., "The Experience of Emergency Department Providers with Embedded Palliative Care During COVID," *Journal of Pain and Symptom Management* 60, no. 5 (2020): E35–E43, https://doi.org/10.1016/j.jpainsymman.2020.08.007.

p. 191 **only one-third of Americans:** Kuldeep N. Yadav, Nicole B. Gabler, Elizabeth Cooney, Saida Kent, Jennifer Kim, Nicole Herbst, Adjoa Mante, Scott D. Halpern, and Katherine R. Courtright, "Approximately One in Three US Adults Completes Any Type of Advance Directive for End-Of-Life Care," *Health Affairs* 36, no. 7 (2017): 1244–1251, https:// doi.org/10.1377/hlthaff.2017.0175.

p. 194 **recipients are white:** "NHPCO Facts and Figures," National Hospice and Palliative Care Organization," August 20, 2020, 10, https://www .nhpco.org/wp-content/uploads/NHPCO-Facts-Figures-2020-edition.pdf.

p. 194 **far below their representation:** "Quick Facts," US Census Bureau, July 1, 2019, https://www.census.gov/quickfacts/fact/table/US/PST045219.

p. 194 **surveyed hospice staff:** Dulce M. Cruz-Oliver and Sandra Sanchez-Reilly, "Barriers to Quality End-of-Life Care for Latinos: Hospice Health Care Professionals' Perspective," *Journal of Hospice & Palliative Nursing* 18, no. 6 (2016): 505–511, https://doi.org/10.1097/NJH.0000000000000277.

p. 194 **created a telenovela:** Dulce M. Cruz-Oliver, Kirsten Ellis, and Sandra Sanchez-Reilly, "Caregivers Like Me: An Education Intervention for Family Caregivers of Latino Elders at End-of-Life," *MedEdPORTAL* 12, no. 10448 (2016), http://doi.org/10.15766/mep_2374-8265.10448.

p. 194 **Black and Hispanic dialysis patients:** Yumeng Wen, "Trends and Racial Disparities of Palliative Care Use among Hospitalized Patients with ESKD on Dialysis," *Journal of the American Society of Nephrology* 30, no. 9 (2019): 1687–1696, https://doi.org/10.1681/ASN.2018121256.

p. 196 **published a qualitative study:** Mary Isaacson, "Addressing Palliative and End-of-Life Care Needs with Native American Elders," *International Journal of Palliative Nursing* 24, no. 4 (2018): 160–168, https://doi.org/10.12968/ijpn.2018.24.4.160.

p. 196 **IHS is severely underfunded:** Sahir Doshi, Allison Jordan, Kate Kelly, and Danyelle Solomon, "The COVID-19 Response in Indian Country," Center for American Progress, June 18, 2020, https://www.americanprogress.org/issues/green/reports/2020/06/18/486480/covid-19-response-indian-country/.

p. 196 **under the Affordable Care Act:** Analyst in Health Services, "Indian Health Care: Impact of the Affordable Care Act (ACA)," Congressional Research Service, January 9, 2014, https://www.everycrsreport.com/reports/R41152.html.

p. 197 **an earlier program:** Mary Isaacson, "Wakani Ewastepikte: An Advance Directive Education Project with American Indian Elders," *Journal of Hospice and Palliative Nursing* 19, no. 6 (2017): 580–587, https://doi.org/10.1097/NJH.0000000000000392.

p. 198 **Medicare began covering:** Wyatt Koma, Juliette Cubanski, and Tricia Neuman, "Medicare and Telehealth: Coverage and Use During the COVID-19 Pandemic and Options for the Future," Kaiser Family Foundation, May 19, 2021, https://www.kff.org/medicare/issue-brief/medicare-and-telehealth-coverage-and-use-during-the-covid-19-pandemic-and-options-for-the-future/.

p. 199 **all sixty-seven counties:** "What Is Rural?" Alabama Rural Health Association, accessed June 1, 2021, https://arhaonline.org/what-is-rural/.

p. 199 **research her colleague:** See Ronit Elk, Alvin Reaves, Karen Jones, Ramona Rhodes, and Wendy Anderson, "Rural African American Pastors' Perspectives on EoL Care for Their Congregants: Phase One of a Three-Phase Pilot Study (SA518A)," *Journal of Pain and Symptom Management* 55, no. 2 (2018): 647, https://doi.org/10.1016/j.jpainsymman.2017.12.192.

p. 200 **finding that palliative care clinicians:** Arif H. Kamal, Janet H. Bull, Steven P. Wolf, Keith M. Swetz, Tait D. Shanafelt, Katherine Ast, Dio Kavakieratos, Christian T. Sinclair, and Amy P. Abernethy, "Prevalence and Predictors of Burnout Among Hospice and Palliative Care Clinicians in the U.S.," *Journal of Pain Symptom Management* 51, no. 4 (2016): 690–696, https://doi.org/10.1016/j.jpainsymman.2015.10.020.

p. 200 **requiring them to retract:** Arif H. Kamal, Janet H. Bull, Steven P. Wolf, Keith M. Swetz, Tait D. Shanafelt, Katherine Ast, Dio Kavakieratos, and Christian T. Sinclair., "Retraction of 'Prevalence and Predictors of Burnout Among Hospice and Palliative Care Professionals From 2016 Apr;51(4): 690–6," *Journal of Pain Symptom Management* 59, no. 5 (2020): 965, https://doi.org/10.1016/j.jpainsymman.2020.03.027.

p. 201 **Kamal's research predicts:** Arif H. Kamal, Steven P. Wolf, Jesse Troy, Victoria Leff, Constance Dahlin, Joseph D. Rotella, George Handzo, Phillip E. Rodgers, and Evan R. Myers, "Policy Changes Key to Promoting Sustainability and Growth of the Specialty Palliative Care Workforce," *Health Affairs* 38, no. 6 (2019): 910–918, https://doi.org/10.1377/hlthaff.2019.00018.

p. 203 **authored a blog:** Stacie Sinclair, "'We Are in a War': Mitigating Burnout in COVID-19," Center to Advance Palliative Care, July 13, 2020, https://www.capc.org/blog/we-are-in-a-war-mitigating-burnout-in-covid-19/.

p. 206 **hospitals involved in palliative care programs:** May Hua, Xiaoyue Ma, R. Sean Morrison, Guohua Li, and Hannah Wunsch, "Association between the Availability of Hospital-based Palliative Care and Treatment Intensity for Critically Ill Patients," *Annals of the American Thoracic Society* 15, no. 9 (2017): 1067–1074, https://doi.org/10.1513/AnnalsATS.201711-872OC.

Chapter 11

p. 210 **wrote of the case:** Timothy Quill, "Death and Dignity—A Case of Individualized Decision-Making," *The New England Journal of Medicine* 324, no. 10 (1991): 691–694, https://doi.org/10.1056/NEJM199103073241010.

p. 210 **Jack Kevorkian:** *Encyclopedia Britannica Online,* s.v. "Jack Kevorkian," updated May 30, 2021, https://www.britannica.com/biography /Jack-Kevorkian.

p. 210 **second-degree murder verdict:** Fred Charatan, "Dr Kevorkian Found Guilty of Second Degree Murder," *British Medical Journal* 318, no. 7189 (1999): 962, https://www.ncbi.nlm.nih.gov/pmc/articles/PMC1174693/.

p. 210 **lead plaintiff in a case:** Vacco v. Quill, 95–1858 U.S. 793 (1997), https://supreme.justia.com/cases/federal/us/521/793/.

p. 210 **eight other states:** "Death with Dignity Acts," Death with Dignity, accessed June 1, 2021, https://deathwithdignity.org/learn/death-with -dignity-acts/.

p. 211 **generally stringent:** "How Death with Dignity Laws Work," Death with Dignity, accessed June 1, 2021, https://deathwithdignity.org/learn/access/.

p. 211 **active euthanasia:** "Euthanasia," Center for Health Ethics, University of Missouri School of Medicine, accessed June 1, 2021, https://medi-cine.missouri.edu/centers-institutes-labs/health-ethics/faq/euthanasia.

p. 211 **legal in the Netherlands:** "The Dutch Termination of Life on Request and Assisted Suicide (Review Procedures) Act," *Ethical Perspectives* 9, no. 2–3 (2002): 176–181, https://doi.org/10.2143/EP.9.2.503855.

p. 212 **a legal complaint:** Cornelius D. Mahoney and Barbara Morris, MD v. Centura Health Corporation, a Colorado non-profit corporation 2019CV31980 U.S. (2019), https://ewscripps.brightspotcdn.com/6d /b8/711cdbad4f899fb998041ca73f78/mahoney-morris-v-centura.pdf.

p. 212 **Centura fired Morris:** "Understanding Centura Health's Position on Colorado EOLOA," Centura Health, accessed June 1, 2021, https:// www.centura.org/patients-and-families/EOLOA.

p. 212 **amended the lawsuit:** Barbara Morris, MD v. Centura Health Corpo-ration, a Colorado non-profit corporation, and Catholic Health Initia-tives Colorado d/b/a Centura Health-St. Anthony Hospital, a Colorado non-profit corporation 2019CV31980 U.S. (2019), http://thaddeuspope .com/images/Centura_-_First_Amended_Complaint_10-07-19.PDF.

p. 212 **commonly used barbiturates:** Jennie Dear, "The Doctors Who Invented a New Way to Help People Die," *Atlantic,* January 22, 2019, https://www.theatlantic.com/health/archive/2019/01/medical-aid-in -dying-medications/580591/.

p. 212 **covered by insurance:** David Grube and Ashley Cardenas, "Insurance Coverage and Aid-in-Dying Medication Costs," *JAMA Oncology* 3, no. 8 (2017): 1137, https://doi.org/10.1001/jamaoncol.2016.6585.

p. 212 **seek other options:** "Death with Dignity: Preparing for the Last Day," End of Life Washington, February 2020, https://endoflifewa.org/wp -content/uploads/2020/02/Preparations-for-the-Last-Day-Feb-2020.pdf.

p. 212 **in rural areas:** Mara Buchbinder, "Access to Aid-in-Dying in the United States: Shifting the Debate from Rights to Justice," *American Journal of Public Health* 108, no. 6 (2018): 754–759, https://doi.org/10.2105 /AJPH.2018.304352.

p. 214 **data from Oregon and Washington:** Luai Al Rabadi, Michael LeBlanc, Taylor Bucy, Lee M. Ellis, Dawn L. Hershman, Frank L. Meyskens Jr., Lynne Taylor, and Charles D. Blanke, "Trends in Medical Aid in Dying in Oregon and Washington," *JAMA Network Open* 2, no. 8 (2019): e198648, https://doi.org/10.1001/jamanetworkopen.2019.8648.

p. 219 **like abortion:** Rachel Hajar, "The Physician's Oath: Historical Perspectives," *Heart Views* 18, no. 4 (2017): 154–159, https://doi.org /10.4103/HEARTVIEWS.HEARTVIEWS_131_17.

p. 220 **well-being at the end of life:** Ira Byock, *The Best Care Possible: A Physician's Quest to Transform Care Through the End of Life* (New York: Avery, 2012), Kindle.

p. 222 **published an article:** Chelsia Danielle Harris, "Physician-Assisted Suicide: A Nurse's Perspective," *Nursing* 44, no. 3 (2014): 55–58, https:// www.doi.org/10.1097/01.NURSE.0000438713.05098.b8.

p. 223 **Oregon's 1999 report:** Arthur E. Chin, Katrina Hedberg, Grant K. Higginson, and Davide W. Fleming, "Legalized Physician-Assisted Suicide in Oregon—The First Year's Experience," *The New England Journal of Medicine* 340, no. 7 (1999): 577–583, https://doi.org/10.1056 /NEJM199902183400724.

p. 223 **series of interviews:** Steven K. Dobscha, Ronald T. Heintz, Nancy Press, and Linda Ganzini, "Oregon Physicians' Responses to Requests for Assisted Suicide: A Qualitative Study," *Journal of Palliative Medicine* 7, no. 3 (2004): 451–461, https://doi.org/10.1089/1096621041349374.

p. 224 **A 2020 analysis:** Joseph G. Barsness, Casey R. Regnier, C. Christopher Hook, and Paul S. Mueller, "US Medical and Surgical Society Position Statements on Physician-Assisted Suicide and Euthanasia: A Review," *BMC Medical Ethics* 21, no. 1 (2020): 111, https://doi.org /10.1186/s12910-020-00556-5.

p. 224 **World Medical Association:** "WMA Declaration on Euthanasia and Physician-Assisted Suicide," World Medical Association, October 2019, https://www.wma.net/policies-post/declaration-on-euthanasia-and -physician-assisted-suicide/.

p. 224 **American Medical Association:** "Physician-Assisted Suicide," American Medical Association, accessed June 1, 2021, https://www.ama-assn.org/delivering-care/ethics/physician-assisted-suicide.

p. 225 **American Nurses Association:** "ANA Advises Objectivity in New Medical Aid in Dying Position," American Nurses Association, June 26, 2019, https://www.nursingworld.org/news/news-releases/2019-news-releases/ana-advises-objectivity-in-new-medical-aid-in-dying-position/.

p. 225 **countries such as Canada:** "Medical Assistance in Dying," Government of Canada, accessed June 1, 2021, https://www.canada.ca/en/health-canada/services/medical-assistance-dying.html.

p. 225 **Hawaii is considering legislation:** "SB839 SD2," Hawaii State Legislature, accessed June 1, 2021, https://www.capitol.hawaii.gov/measure_indiv.aspx?billtype=SB&billnumber=839&year=2021.

p. 225 **In a 2017 paper:** Felicia Stokes, "The Emerging Role of Nurse Practitioners in Physician-Assisted Death," *The Journal for Nurse Practitioners* 13, no. 2 (2017): 150–155, https://doi.org/10.1016/j.nurpra.2016.08.029.

Chapter 12

p. 236 **volunteers in hospitals:** Renee Brent Hotchkiss, Lynn Unruh, and Myron D. Fottler, "The Role, Measurement, and Impact of Volunteerism in Hospitals," *Nonprofit and Voluntary Sector Quarterly* 43, no. 6 (2014): 1111–1128, https://doi.org/10.1177/0899764014549057.

p. 238 **a core nursing skill:** Kathryn Westman and Cathy Blaisdell, "Many Benefits, Little Risk: The Use of Massage in Nursing Practice," *American Journal of Nursing* 116, no. 1 (2016): 34–39, https://doi.org/10.1097/01.NAJ.0000476164.97929.f2.

p. 241 **many physicians have identified:** John Campanelli, "The Benefits of Physician Volunteering," Medical Economics, July 25, 2017, https://www.medicaleconomics.com/view/benefits-physician-volunteering.

p. 242 **rainy night in Oregon:** Sandra Clarke, "No One Dies Alone," How We Die, accessed June 1, 2021, http://www.how-we-die.org/HowWeDie/story?sid=8.

p. 242 **Mayo Clinic video:** Mayo Clinic, "The Birth of 'No One Dies Alone,'" You Tube video, 1:42, October 10, 2013, https://www.youtube.com/watch?v=zHbQwHHR7WI.

p. 247 **a study:** Anita Catlin, Michael Cobbina, Raymond Dougherty, and Denise Laws, "Music, Spirituality, and Caring Science: The Effect of *a Cappella* Song on Healthcare Staff in Medical-Surgical Units,"

International Journal for Human Caring 23, no. 3 (2019): 234–241,
https://doi.org/10.20467/1091-5710.23.3.234.

Conclusion

p. 249 **first COVID-19 cases:** AJMC Staff, "A Timeline of COVID-19 Developments in 2020," *The American Journal of Managed Care,* January 1, 2021, https://www.ajmc.com/view/a-timeline-of-covid19-developments-in-2020.

p. 249 **more than half a million deaths:** COVID Data Tracker, Centers for Disease Control and Prevention, accessed June 1, 2021, https://covid.cdc.gov/covid-data-tracker/#datatracker-home.

p. 249 **reductions in income:** Susan Ladika, "The Pandemic One Year In: Providers Struggle with Loss of Revenue," Managed Healthcare Executive, March 10, 2021, https://www.managedhealthcareexecutive.com/view/the-pandemic-one-year-in-providers-struggle-with-loss-of-revenue.

p. 249 **Many were warned:** Olivia Carville, Emma Court, and Kristen V. Brown, "Hospitals Tell Doctors They'll Be Fired If They Speak Out about Lack of Gear," Bloomberg, March 31, 2020, https://www.bloomberg.com/news/articles/2020-03-31/hospitals-tell-doctors-they-ll-be-fired-if-they-talk-to-press.

p. 249 **Lorna Breen:** Shannon Firth, "Dr. Lorna Breen Bill to Prevent Provider Suicide Reintroduced in Congress," Medpage Today, March 5, 2021, https://www.medpagetoday.com/publichealthpolicy/healthpolicy/91510.

p. 250 **an annual increase:** Ryan Basen, "It's Official: Med School Applications Well Up This Cycle," Medpage Today, January 7, 2021, https://www.medpagetoday.com/publichealthpolicy/medicaleducation/90581.

p. 250 **to relaxed criteria:** Patrick Thomas, "U.S. Medical School Applications Soar in Covid-19 Era," *Wall Street Journal,* September 21, 2020, https://www.wsj.com/articles/u-s-medical-school-applications-soar-in-covid-19-era-11600688871.

p. 250 **minority populations:** Leo Lopez III, Louis H. Hart III, and Mitchell H. Katz, "Racial and Ethnic Health Disparities Related to COVID-19," *Journal of the American Medical Association* 325, no. 8 (2021): 719–720, https://doi.org/10.1001/jama.2020.26443.

p. 250 **Asian Americans:** "Covid-19 Fueling Anti-Asian Racism and Xenophobia Worldwide," Human Rights Watch, May 12, 2020, https://www.hrw.org/news/2020/05/12/covid-19-fueling-anti-asian-racism-and-xenophobia-worldwide.

p. 250 **less visible frontline workers:** Danielle Renwick and Shoshana Dubnow, "Exclusive: Over 900 Health Workers Have Died of COVID-19. And the Toll Is Rising," *The Guardian* and Kaiser Health News, August 11, 2020, https://khn.org/news/exclusive-over-900-health-workers-have -died-of-covid-19-and-the-toll-is-rising/.

p. 250 **other forms:** Yea-Hung Chen, Maria Glymour, Alicia Riley, John Balmes, Kate Duchowny, Robert Harrison, Ellicott Matthay, and Kirsten Bibbins-Domingo, "Excess Mortality Associated with the COVID-19 Pandemic among Californians 18-65 Years of Age, by Occupational Sector and Occupation: March through October 2020," medRxiv, January 22, 2021, https://doi.org/10.1101/2021.01.21.21250266.

p. 250 **Medicare Trust Fund:** "The Outlook for Major Federal Trust Funds: 2020 to 2030," Congressional Budget Office, September 2020, p. 2, https://www.cbo.gov/system/files/2020-09/56523-Trust-Funds.pdf.

p. 250 **3,000 healthcare professionals:** "Lost on the Frontline," *The Guardian* and Kaiser Health News, accessed June 1, 2021, https://www.theguardian .com/us-news/ng-interactive/2020/aug/11/lost-on-the-frontline-covid -19-coronavirus-us-healthcare-workers-deaths-database.

p. 252 **a 2021 survey found:** "Your Patients Are Ready," VITAS Healthcare, accessed June 1, 2021, https://www.vitas.com/for-healthcare -professionals/education-and-training/talking-to-your-patients-about -end-of-life.

p. 252 **an increase of 24 percent:** "Most Americans 'Relieved' to Talk about End-of-Life Care," The Conversation Project, April 10, 2018, https:// theconversationproject.org/wp-content/uploads/2018/07/Final-2018 -Kelton-Findings-Press-Release.pdf.

Index

B

babies
cuddlers, 240–241
portrait sessions, 244–245
Project Knitwell, 117
stillbirth, xiii–xv
Bachl, Karla, 231, 243–244
Back, Anthony, 37–38, 106
balance, 132–138
Bana, Lufta, 96–97
Bartels, Jonathan, 90–91
Bay Area End of Life Options, 213
BEHAVE Wellness, 63
Bickford, Lara, 134–135
Bishop, Lori, 172
*Black Man in a White Coat: A Doctor's
Reflections on Race and Medicine*
(Tweedy), 72
Blanke, Charles, 215–217, 219
Bledsoe, Gregory, 50, 53–54, 57
*The Body Keeps the Score: Brain, Mind, and
the Body in the Healing of Trauma* (van
der Kolk), 166
brain death, 188
brain injuries
caring for unconscious patients, 159
coma treatment strategies, 160–161
connecting with patients'
families, 160
extracorporeal membrane
oxygenation (ECMO), 161–162
personhood, 153–159
Breen, Lorna, 249
Bresnahan, Linda, 99
Brown, Brené, 145
Buffington, Mary, 67–68, 72–73
Bullock, Karen, 195–196
bullying, 57–63
Bunge, Kristen, 11, 24
burnout, 65–73
definition of, 66
female physicians, 71–72
The Healer's Art course, 111–112
hospice workers, 171
Maslach Burnout Inventory (MBI),
105, 109
minorities in academia, 72
minority groups, 72

nurses, 9, 66–68
OB-GYNs, 71
palliative care providers, 200–204
physicians, 8–9, 71–72, 80
PTSD, 67
reading for pleasure, 113–114
recognition/ability to be heard, 235
residents, 8
self-care, 109–110
Stanford Model of Professional
Fulfillment, 112
students, 106, 109
studies, 105–106
urologists, 69–70
work-life balance, 132–138
Burnout Ward, 73
Byock, Ira, 219–220

C

cadavers
dissection, 11–12
writing obituaries for, 113
California nurse-patient ratios during
Covid-19 pandemic, 68
Campbell, Robert Chodo, 95
cancer patients
delivering bad news, 36
"the ones that should never have
happened", 29
Caparosa, Carol, 116–117
Caputo-Seidler, Jennifer, 31–33,
39–40, 46
Cárdenas, Caroline, 125–126, 138–139
Caregivers Like Me (Cuidadores Como Yo)
telenovela, 194
Carter's Quiet Care Cuddlers, 240–241
Cassell, Joan, 59
Centers for Disease Control and
Prevention (CDC) causes of death
statistics, 88
Centura Health Corporation, 212
certified music practitioners, 236, 237
certified nursing assistants (CNAs),
175–176, 229–230
recognition/ability to be heard, 235
Cesarz, Alison, 16
chaplains, 90, 92–98
Charon, Rita, 140

Niebuhr, Shelly, 236–237
NMA (National Medical Association),
      152
No One Dies Alone (NODA) program,
      242, 243, 244
nonclinical staff, 230–241. *See also*
      volunteers
nonmedical modalities, hospice
      patients, 181
Now I Lay Me Down to Sleep
      (NILMDTS) program, 244–245
Nuland, Sherwin, 7
Numann, Patricia, 27–28, 31, 35
numbing, 89
nurse-patient ratios, 68–69
nurses
      assisted dying, 214, 225–226
      bullying, 59–60
      burnout, 9, 66–68
      ICU, 121
      need for self-care, 21–25
      palliative care strain on clinicians,
            192–193
      PTSD, 9, 66–67
      retreats, 121–122
      The Sacred Art of Nursing
            workshops, 120
      shortage of, 69
      suicide, 9
      trust, 146
nursing assistants (CNAs), 175–176,
      229–230, 235
nursing homes during COVID-19
      pandemic, 49, 175
Nursing Practice: The Ethical Issues
      (Jameton), 45
nursing students, depression, 8

O

O'Rourke, Mark, 220–221
Obayuwana, Alphonsus, 137–138
OB-GYN burnout, 71, 95
obituaries for cadavers, 113
Ofri, Danielle, xiii–xv, 77
Olson, DaiWai, 159–161
On Death and Dying (Kübler-Ross), 2, 170
oncology nurses, retreats with cancer
      survivors, 121–122

operating room environment, 58–61
opioids, 82–83, 149
organ donors, 91
Ortenzio, Lou, 82–83
Overcash, Janine, 30, 36
overdose, 104
Owen, Adrian, 153–154, 160–161
Owen, Mary, 43–44, 46

P

pain management, 202
palliative care, 187–189
      access to, 190, 193–200
      advance directives, 191–192
      burnout, 200–204
      chaplains, 204–205
      coining of term "palliative care", 189
      COVID-19 pandemic, 191
      disenfranchised communities,
            194–199
      end-of-life documents, 191–192
      goals-of-care conversations, 163,
            187–189, 204
      ICU and ER, 206–207
      inclusion of family and pastoral
            care, 199
      Latino patients and their
            caregivers, 194
      moral distress, 206
      moral injury, 201
      patient memorial events, 193
      racial inequity, 194–196
      serious illness patients, 189–190
      social workers, 202–203
      strain on clinicians, 192–193
      teams of care providers, 188–207
      telehealth, 198–199, 203
      underserved areas, 194, 196–200
      wellness debriefings, 205–206
panic attacks, 67–68
Pantilat, Steven, 189–190, 193, 198
Pape, Theresa Bender, 154–156, 160
paramedics and EMTs
      calling deaths in the field, 38–39
      suicide, 80–82
      trauma, 10
PAS (physician-assisted suicide), 217. *See
      also* assisted dying

traumatic brain injuries
    caring for unconscious patients, 159
    coma treatment strategies, 160–161
    connecting with patients' families, 160
    extracorporeal membrane
        oxygenation (ECMO), 161–162
    personhood, 153–159
Traywick, Joey, 163–166
trust. *See also* connection
    2020 Gallup poll, 146
    Black community, 151–152
    establishing, 146–153
Trzeciak, Stephen, 128, 131
Tweedy, Damon, 72

U

unconscious patients
    caring for, 159
    coma treatment strategies, 160–161
    connecting with patients'
        families, 160
    extracorporeal membrane
        oxygenation (ECMO), 161–162
    personhood, 153–159
Uniform Determination of Death Act in
    1981, 188
University of New Mexico writing
    retreat, 122
urologist burnout, 69–70

V

VA hospice, 181
vaccines, and patient trust, 151–152
value-based care, 150
van der Kolk, Bessel, 166
Verghese, Danielle, 13–14, 20–21
Viner, Edward, 131
Virginia Health Practitioners
    Monitoring Program (HPMP), 79
Virkstis, Katherine, 143
VitalTalk, 37
Vitez, Michael, 140–141
Viviano, Julianne, 48–49, 65–67
voluntary stopping eating and drinking
    (VSED), 226
volunteers, 230–248
    COVID-19 pandemic, 231
    cuddlers, 240–241
    massage therapists, 237–238

medical interpreters, 231–234
music therapists, 236–237
No One Dies Alone (NODA),
    242–244
Now I Lay Mé Down to Sleep
    (NILMDTS) portraits, 244–245
pet therapy, 238–240
Reading with Royalty, 240
Threshold Choir, 246–247
VSED (voluntary stopping eating and
    drinking), 226

W

Wald, Florence, 170
Warraich, Haider, 145–150
Weinstein, Michael, 83–84
Weller, Francis, 87
wellness debriefings, 205–206
wellness retreats, 118, 122–123
Welzant, Victor, 102–104
West, Colin, 105–106
*When We Do Harm: A Doctor Confronts
    Medical Error* (Ofri), 77
Whitman, Walt, 115
Wible, Pamela, 80, 99, 122–124
WMA. *See* World Medical Association
    (WMA)
The Woman in the Surgeon's Body (Cassell),
    59
Wong Gregorio, Ilene, 70–71
work-life balance, 132–138
workplace violence, 52–57
workshops, 119–121
    AWARE, 108
    writing, 139–140
World Medical Association (WMA)
    Declaration of Geneva, 19
    opposition to MAID/PAS, 224
writing, 139–143
    journaling, 33
    patient's stories, 139–140
    writing retreat, 122
Wu, Albert, 74–75

Z

Zen Center for Contemplative Care, 95
Zenger, Brian, 242–243
Zerwas, Stephanie, 100–101
Zitter, Jessica, 88–89, 92

Acknowledgments

First and foremost, I would like to thank the numerous healthcare workers—doctors, nurses, EMTs, CNAs, medical interpreters, volunteers, and others—who shared their very personal stories. Many took time out of hectic schedules during a global pandemic to do so, often due to a strong belief in the need for this book. I'm beyond grateful for their openness and bravery, and for the trust they granted me. I hope that I have done them justice.

Shayna Keyles, my editor at North Atlantic Books, had the prescient vision to solicit this work just when it would be most needed. She has served as a guiding light throughout the process, and her thoughtful suggestions have been essential to shaping complex subject matter into a cohesive story. To North Atlantic Books' design team, which came up with the beautiful cover; its marketing team; and the many others who have supported this project from behind the scenes: thank you. I'm immensely grateful to Suzette Sherman and Kathleen Clohessy at SevenPonds for their sage guidance on the 2019 article that became the springboard for this book ("New Rituals Lessen Trauma of Code Blue Deaths for Clinicians"), as well as for Suzette's kind permission to reprint portions of that text in Chapters 2 and 5.

This book could not have been completed on time without generous support from the Alfred P. Sloan Foundation Program in Public Understanding of Science and Technology, which not only provided funds that enabled me to set aside other projects and focus on the task at hand, but also for a foreword writer and two manuscript reviewers. I am indebted to LaTonya Trotter for her wise, far-reaching insight, and to Yangyang

Deng for his keen eye for detail. Meanwhile, Danielle Ofri has been kind enough to pen an incredible foreword, blending her medical knowledge and literary talent to offer a touching firsthand perspective. As a writer who does not practice medicine, I appreciate her very personal contribution regarding the widespread impact of grief and trauma in the field.

I'm deeply grateful to Columbia University's Graduate School of Journalism, and to the mentors who have nurtured and supported me throughout my career. In particular, Joshua Friedman, Michael Shapiro, and Mike Hoyt have been essential to making me the reporter and writer I am today. I would like to thank the Logan Nonfiction Program for their Spring 2021 virtual fellowship, and the professional development, camaraderie, and support provided by a community of talented fellows. Mark Bowden's insightful commentary was particularly helpful in fine-tuning this manuscript.

Writing is a solitary endeavor, and I'm thankful for the strong backing of friends and family, who—near and, most often, far—provided companionship, encouragement, and unfailing support during this process. For my parents and sisters, who have been formative influences in my early years of reading and writing, and who have always provided a warm place to come home to. For my Lewis & Clark College crew, which has been such a longstanding, deeply treasured, and often necessary foundation of grounding and belonging in my life. For Abraham Daniel and his lovely family in Chennai, India, where the bulk of this book was written. For Jose, Alejandro, and others whose friendship provided a welcome distraction, however briefly, from the arduous task at hand. And for those sisters of my soul: Vera, Bree, Crystal, Cheri, Shelly, and those I have yet to meet. I can't imagine navigating this journey of life without you.

A book is nothing without readers, and so I would like to thank each and every person who has taken the time to read this book. I hope you have found these healthcare workers' stories as profound and influential as I have, and that they inspire hope and positive change in supporting clinicians and patients alike.

About the Author

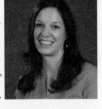

RACHEL JONES is a freelance writer whose nonfiction has appeared in *Time* magazine, *The Lancet*, *The Delacorte Review*, *Scientific American*, *The Antigonish Review*, *Columbia Journalism Review*, and many other publications. She obtained a BA in sociology and studio art from Lewis & Clark College in Portland, Oregon. After earning her MS from Columbia University's Graduate School of Journalism, Rachel spent more than four years as a reporter in Caracas, Venezuela, including a year and a half as a correspondent for The Associated Press. More recently, she has been exploring a longstanding interest in death and dying as a staff writer for SevenPonds, a website and online magazine that informs the public about a wide array of issues related to end of life. Jones is the recipient of a Pulitzer traveling fellowship and an Overseas Press Club Foundation scholarship. You can learn more about her work at rachelevangelinejones.com.

About North Atlantic Books

North Atlantic Books (NAB) is a 501(c)(3) nonprofit publisher committed to a bold exploration of the relationships between mind, body, spirit, culture, and nature. Founded in 1974, NAB aims to nurture a holistic view of the arts, sciences, humanities, and healing. To make a donation or to learn more about our books, authors, events, and newsletter, please visit www.northatlanticbooks.com.